40 DAYS TO RESET YOUR LIFE

APPLYING GOD'S WISDOM FOR PHYSICAL AND SPIRITUAL RENEWAL

SHANE IDLEMAN

EL PASEO PUBLICATIONS

Copyright © 2021 Shane Idleman

All rights reserved. No part of this publication may be reproduced or distributed in any form or by any means or stored in a database or retrieval system without prior written permission from the publisher and/or author.

Published by El Paseo Publications.

Printed in the United States of America.

Scripture is taken from the New King James Version®. Copyright © 1982 by Thomas Nelson. Used by permission. All rights reserved. Scriptures and quotes within quotation marks are exact quotes; whereas, paraphrased Scriptures and quotes are often italicized.

Scripture quotations marked (NIV) are taken from the Holy Bible, New International Version®, NIV®. Copyright © 1973, 1978, 1984, 2011 by Biblica, Inc.™ Used by permission of Zondervan. All rights reserved worldwide. www.zondervan.com The "NIV" and "New International Version" are trademarks registered in the United States Patent and Trademark Office by Biblica, Inc.™

Scripture quotations marked (NASB) are taken from the New American Standard Bible® (NASB), Copyright © 1960, 1962, 1963, 1968, 1971, 1972, 1973, 1975, 1977, 1995 by The Lockman Foundation. Used by permission: www.Lockman.org.

ISBN-13: 978-1-7343774-2-2

Cover photo provided by *Gallery 158, Photos* by Tom Okeefe. Interior design by Steve Bremner, initial editing by Christine Ramsey, and cover by Lena DeYoung.

ACKNOWLEDGMENTS

A special thanks to my mom, Diane Idleman, who passed away in September 2020. She would have loved the book cover that we chose; it was one of her favorite vacation spots. She had been my main editor since 2000. God used her in a powerful way to help spread the message of hope and truth.

And special thanks to my wife, Morgan, who is always helpful, encouraging, and supportive when it comes to writing another book. Thank you to my five kids as well—you're such a blessing.

DISCLAIMER

This book was written based on personal experience and observation as well as many outside reputable resources. *If professional assistance is needed, the services of a capable authority are recommended.* The views expressed in this book should not replace professional medical advice. Readers should seek medical supervision before starting or altering a dietary plan, including fasting.

Links to resources, articles, and videos are provided for e-book users (you must be online for this feature to work). If you're reading the printed version of this book, you may want to consider downloading the ebook version so that you can access the links. The links are current up to the printing date. Neither the publisher nor the author assumes responsibility for errors or changes that occur after publication. Additionally, although books, articles, and videos are recommended, the author doesn't necessarily agree with every view.

The exact source of some of the quotes is unknown, but most of them are well known and used often in Christian literature. We are also hoping to make the audible version of this book available soon.

"The evidence of being a Christian is not that there are no tactical defeats in the war, but that you keep fighting till the promised victory is given."[1]

CONTENTS

Acknowledgments	iii
Disclaimer	1
Epigraph 1	3
Epigraph 2	9
Introduction . . . Start Here	11

PART ONE
BUILDING THE FOUNDATION

What is a Reset?	21
Focus on Progress, not Perfection	27
Why Forty and Why Fasting?	33
Fasting Applies Pressure to the Spiritual Realm	39
Be on Guard in These Two Areas	45
Stimulants—Robbing Peter and Plundering Paul	49
If You Fail, Fall Forward	53
What Type of Fast Should I Do?	57
The Hardest Part of a Fast	69
Biblically Speaking, What Should I Eat?	79
A Must-Read Fasting Experience	89
The Power of the Made-Up Mind	99

PART TWO
DAILY REFLECTIONS

1. How to Rest in Turbulent Times	103
2. Are You Spiritually Healthy?	105
3. How Are You Measuring Success?	107
4. Why Have I Lost My Passion For Life?	109
5. What Goes In Comes Out	113
6. Truth–A Hill on Which to Die	117
7. The Desperate Need For Genuine Worship	119
8. Worship—The Thermometer of the Heart	123
9. The Beginning of Wisdom and Knowledge	125

10. Why Doesn't Success Satisfy?	129
11. Resetting Your Site on the Target	133
12. This Word Will Set You Free	137
13. Experiencing God Through His Spirit	141
14. Men—Life is a Battleground, Not a Playground	145
15. The Difference Between Happiness and Joy	149
16. Money—Servant or Master?	153
17. Experiencing God Through Holiness	157
18. Is The World Infecting You?	161
19. God's Will is Always Right on Time	165
20. The Cost of Speaking the Truth	169
21. I'm Too Busy to Pray	173
22. Avoid These Three Destructive Influences	177
23. The Sinful Nature is at War with God	181
24. Understanding Temptation	185
25. Hope For The Hurting	189
26. Understanding Grace	193
27. A Word To The Critical Heart	197
28. Prone to Wander - Lord I Feel it	201
29. The Cure For Doubt And Fear	205
30. Are You On The Verge Of Wrecking Your Life?	209
31. There Is Another in the Fire with You	213
32. Seven Tips for Turbulent Times	217
33. Is Your Blessing Waiting on You?	221
34. Five Ways to Prevail in Prayer	225
35. Traits of False Prophets	229
36. Traits of False Prophets	233
37. Dealing with Depression and Mental Illness	237
38. Microwave Christianity Isn't Healthy	241
39. Surviving the Anointing	245
40. Why Revival is America's Only Hope!	249
Appendix: My Daily Fasting Breakdown	255
My Top Ten Health Tips	259
Daily Checklist	261
Recommended Reading	263

Other Books By The Author 265
Notes 269

"You have not sought the Lord with *'your whole heart'* until you have tried a protracted season of prayer and fasting. Many Christians have been praying for years about certain problems. Sometimes these prayers are not answered."

"But in many cases, where fasting has been added to the prayers, along with deep consecration and weeping before God, the answer has miraculously come to hand."

- Gordon Cove

INTRODUCTION... START HERE

A very high percentage of people quit a few weeks after beginning a new endeavor because the results they had hoped for take longer than planned.

Although this book is focused primarily on building spiritual health, we shouldn't overlook physical health. In most cases, we can't neglect one and expect the other to flourish. For example, are you filled with love and joy when you keep caving into destructive habits? Are you excited to take care of your body when you keep falling short spiritually? Of course not. The spiritual and the physical are interwoven: "If you don't believe me, spend a week sleeping no more than four or five hours a night and eating nothing but junk food and see how it affects your walk with the Lord, your emotions, and your ability to handle life's problems" (Joel R. Beeke and Nick Thompson).[1]

A SPIRITUAL RESET

As a nation, it's clear that we are dying spiritually. Just look at the media choices that fill our homes, the sexual perversion that runs rampant, and the disdain for God that saturates every fabricate of society, not to mention the catastrophic legislation that is governing our nation. Do we really think that we can mock God in these areas and expect His blessings? No, we cannot. We must realize just how far we have drifted from Him and turn back. We need a spiritual reset.

A PHYSICAL RESET

A few years ago, I challenged people with this statement when I released my book, *HELP! I'm Addicted*: "We are at the crossroads: Opioid and alcohol abuse are leaving a path of destruction in their wake. Obesity is skyrocketing and plaguing millions—it has even reached epidemic levels in children. Cancer and heart disease are the number one killers in America. And on and on it goes from nicotine to caffeine to food—as a society, we are out of control." Little has changed . . . if anything, we are worse off today.

Sadly, most people spend the last decade or two of their lives dying rather than living—confined to homes, frequenting hospitals, and depending on others. As a pastor visiting hospitals and hospital homes, I see firsthand the devastating and debilitating results of poor health choices. Sooner or later, these choices catch up to us.

In the last two decades, the diet industry has tripled its gross annual income to approximately $60 billion[2] with a success rate of only 5% to 10% (depending on what study you read). Did you catch that? We spend $60 billion annually to receive a 5% to 10% return.

Ironically, just before I released this book a thought-provoking article was released titled: *44% of older millennials already have a chronic health condition. Here's what that means for their futures.* Clearly, it's time for a physical reset as well.

When I was in the fitness industry, I witnessed first-hand the devastating effects of everything from childhood obesity and diabetes to every diet-related disease imaginable. In many cases, kids as young as ten years old were forty or fifty pounds overweight. Parents, we are setting them up for failure before their life has even really begun. Even if your kids are not overweight, the massive amounts of sugar and junk food will eventually take its toll on their health. Shouldn't we do more?

Admittedly, there are those who, through no fault of their own, have a debilitating illness or a unique situation that prevents change. I'm assuming that the reader understands that I'm talking to those who *can* make changes.

FASTING AND THE FARMER

Fasting is like a farmer who takes a barren and rundown stretch of wilderness and works hard to transform it into a beautiful garden.

One day, a pastor walks by and comments on the extraordinary beauty of the garden. The farmer replies, "Thank you! I did it all by myself." To that, the pastor responds, "Oh, no sir. You also had the Lord's help."

The farmer shot back, "Well, all right then . . . the Lord did help, but you should have seen it when He was managing it by Himself."

We chuckle, but the principle is profound. Health, like beauty, can flourish when the right environment is created. God gives us all the necessary ingredients, but it's up to us to steward His creation.³ Fasting is one such ingredient.

THE FOUR SUPPORT BEAMS

As a result of everything mentioned above, my focus will be on four support beams—*nutrient-dense nutrition, restorative rest, minimizing stress, and building intimacy with God.* The first part of this book builds with information, motivation, and application, whereas the last two-thirds contain *daily reflections.*

The daily reflections are portions of articles that I've written over the years. Their focus is mainly on intimacy with God, holiness, spiritual disciplines, and repentance. Read one reflection a day and apply it until it becomes a habit. For those who may want to share the *daily reflections* or make copies, many can be found at *ShaneIdleman.com.* Simply type the title into the search bar and click *Go.*

To be clear: Everything pales in comparison to our relationship with God; it holds everything together. Change begins when we stop "doing" and turn everything over to God, admitting that we cannot change in our own strength. We can do nothing without Him (cf. John 15:7). We must build our life on His foundation.

MOTIVATIONAL TIPS

Not surprisingly, a very high percentage of people quit a few weeks after beginning a health endeavor because the results they had hoped for take longer than planned. For this reason, this resource is focused on the long-haul, not the quick fix. It's designed to help maintain motivation during the process, and beyond. Don't become impatient, change takes time.

Here are some tips that will help:

1) Your first tip is to highlight motivational quotes and inspirational facts as you read. Refer to them often. Motivation, like your body, needs constant fuel.

2) Your second tip is to listen to the embedded videos and read the articles in the footnotes. As stated earlier, you must be online for this feature to work. If you're reading the printed version, my encouragement is to also download the ebook in order to access the links. Again, although I recommend resources, I don't necessarily agree with everything they say or promote: *Eat the meat and throw out the bones.*

3) Your third tip is to educate yourself about the lost discipline of fasting. *The difficulty of fasting proves the value of fasting.* "In early church history, fasting was considered one of the pillars of the Christian religion. When the church had [spiritual] power, fasting was an essential part of the faith. Fasting is not mere abstinence from food or from any other pleasure, but is abstinence with a purpose" (Gordon Cove).[4]

ADDITIONAL ENCOURAGEMENT

For added encouragement on fasting, I included a recommended reading list in the back of this book. My book, *Feasting and Fasting*, also answers many questions about fasting that aren't answered in this resource. I also included a link in the footnote to my teachings on fasting as well as a link to healthy menu options and our church's *Healthy Living Support* page.[5]

You can also *subscribe* to my YouTube in the footnote and receive weekly videos covering everything from nutrition to fasting and from theology to Christian living. While there, scroll through older videos and find topics that interest you.[6]

There are highs and lows when fasting. One minute you are motivated and happy, and ten minutes later you are sad and ready to quit. When this happens, ask yourself how you will feel if you don't see this through and succeed. Commitment and perseverance are vital to success. Attitude about life's setbacks and not the setbacks themselves determine success or failure.

Throughout the book, I write about *falling forward*. I'm not encouraging people to blow it; instead, I'm offering hope. It's been well said that everyone we meet is facing a battle that we don't know anything about. Many reading this right now are no doubt facing such challenges. They need encouragement and grace to push through. That's my goal.

Are you ready for a spiritual and physical reset? If so, I'm ready to help.

Special Note: I released a booklet simultaneously with this one. The title is, *Oh God, Would You Rend the Heavens?—Understanding and Contending for a Genuine Spiritual Awakening.* This resource is for those desiring a renewed passion for God—see the section, *Other Books by the Author,* for more information.

Although my books are on many different platforms, you can also access free downloads of the PDFs at ShaneIdleman.com.

For those who prefer listening rather than reading, I'm hoping to release the audio version of this book some time in the future on platforms such as Audible, iTunes, Amazon, etc. My goal is to also offer it free on my website with the ebooks.

The audiobook will give me freedom to elaborate on many of the topics. It will also contain bonus material and added encouragement and motivation for the journey.

PART ONE

BUILDING THE FOUNDATION

WHAT IS A RESET?

During times of crisis, the power of prayer and fasting leads to wisdom, peace, protection, insight, and guidance.

The term *reset* has been thrown around a lot lately. Whether it's a global reset, a financial reset, or a health reset, it's clear that we are intrigued with starting over. The definition of reset, from a biblical standpoint, is *spiritual renewal*. It occurs when people turn back to God and experience Him in profound ways. Thank God for second, third, and fourth chances.

Sadly, we often measure success by how much we *have* or what we *do*, but God looks at our spiritual condition via a broken and contrite heart (cf. Psalm 51:17). Seeking God through fasting, prayer, worship, humility, and obedience must be a priority if we are to experience a true *spiritual* reset: "But those who wait on the LORD shall renew their strength; they shall mount up with wings like eagles, they shall run and not be weary, they shall walk and not faint" (Isaiah 40:31).

I am concerned that many are fearful but not repentant, anxious but not surrendered to God, worried but not worshipful, confused but not diligently seeking Him. What will it take to draw us back to God? We must change course. God hears the prayers of His people and desires to pour out His Spirit on a dry and thirsty land (cf. Joel 2:25-32). Are you dry? Are you thirsty for more of God? Hunger for God leads to a spiritual reset.

THE POWER OF PRAYER AND FASTING

During times of crisis, the power of prayer *and* fasting leads to wisdom, protection, insight, repentance, and guidance. Granted, we can't dismiss God's sovereignty by putting too much emphasis on our effort. But it's clear that spiritual disciplines (with the right heart), can usher in God's blessings, protection, guidance, and provision. For example, look at the cure for judgment that God gave the prophet Joel. Fasting was an important part of it: "Consecrate a fast, call a sacred assembly; gather the elders and all the inhabitants of the land into the house of the Lord your God, and cry out to the Lord" (v. 14). The same call went out to the city of Nineveh in the book of Jonah.

Fasting is also an important spiritual discipline. Jesus said, "when you fast," not "if you fast" (Matthew 6:16). Therefore, my goal going forward is to help you incorporate the discipline of fasting into your life.

Unbeknownst to most people, in addition to the health benefits of fasting, fasting is one of the greatest ways to remove destructive habits and transform your mind with the truth (cf. Romans 12). When fasting, you're also encouraged to be very selective with your thought life and media choices. Instead, use the extra time to read and meditate on God's Word. "We overeat, and then we are too sluggish to pray, and hence we never come within the range of the Spirit, where He can do great things for us and through us" (Gordon Cove).[1] I can definitely relate. *Having a full stomach makes preaching difficult, prayer hard, and worship challenging.* That's why the best time for me to pray, worship, and read the Word is early in the morning on an empty stomach.

FASTING IS A HEART ISSUE

On certain days you may not *feel* like seeking God, but it's not about how you *feel*, it's about aligning your heart with God's. "If I throw out a boat hook from the boat and catch hold of the shore and pull, do I pull the shore to me, or do I pull myself to the shore? Prayer is not pulling God to my will, but the aligning of my will to the will of God" (E. Stanley Jones).[2] Fasting is all about delayed gratification.

The key is to keep moving forward despite feelings: "Now faith is the substance of things hoped for, the evidence of things not seen" (Hebrews 11:1). Genuine faith moves forward despite setbacks, and trusts in God regardless of how we feel. But if you fall, immediately get back up and continue the journey—*fail forward*. For example, if you watch something that you shouldn't, or cave in when fasting, repent and get back on track. Life is a marathon, not a sprint. *I'm not offering a license to sin, I'm offering grace to finish the journey.*

There are times when you may need to even reset your reset. For example, if you're doing well on a fast, but succumb to temptation in a moment of weakness, simply start up again and reset. This humbling process works wonders when it comes to softening the heart.

As Christians, we know that spiritual warfare is very real. The enemy attempts to derail us at every turn. He wants us to quit rather than to build the spiritual muscle of perseverance. *Perseverance is strengthened in the furnace of affliction and in the midst of defeat. It means to stay the course despite difficulties, obstacles, and discouragement.* When we continue down the road, even after crashing, we develop perseverance and fortitude. This is why I often encourage people to use failure as a stepping stone rather than a stumbling block.

I'm also not suggesting that fasting, or fasting for a certain amount of time, is the only way to succeed. God blesses a broken and contrite heart, not a *work* or a timetable. But fasting has been an important spiritual discipline throughout church history, as well as in both the Old and New Testaments. If God is leading you to fast, whether it's short-term or long-term, it's always best to listen and obey. He blesses choices that are focused on Him. This is an important part of the reset.

If you decide to fast, read Isaiah 58 on the importance of having the right heart toward God and others when you fast. It's crucial to maintain thankfulness despite how you feel. There have been times when I entered a fast begrudgingly instead of with joy. I prayed, "Lord, I'm excited to spend this time with you during my fast," but I would complain during the difficult days.

A CHANGED HEART CHANGES HABITS

How bad do you want to reset your life? Will you turn to God with all your heart? Will you humble yourself and repent?

We have become comfortable. All-night prayer meetings have been exchanged for all-night Netflix binges. Powerful worship services where the Spirit of God is moving have been turned into 60-minute programs designed to entertain rather than convict.

We are measuring success by "likes" and "followers" rather than Christlikeness and following Him.

If we have any hope of a spiritual reset, it will begin with a revived heart, and that will come at a price. We must deny ourselves and fully surrender our lives to Christ (cf. Matthew 16). Fasting is an important tool of surrender that meets the requirements of 2 Chronicles 7:14—to humble ourselves, pray, seek God, and turn from sin. Fasting, in a sense, breaks the prideful heart into pieces.

A changed heart changes habits. It all begins here.

FOCUS ON PROGRESS, NOT PERFECTION

Use failure as a stepping stone rather than a stumbling block. View fasting as planting seeds rather than consuming fruit.

Very few can fast or eat perfectly, and none of us can live perfectly. It's much easier to rest and fast if we have no responsibilities, sleep often, and remove all food items within a five-mile radius, but that's not practical for many of us. Although fasting and healthy eating retreats are great, most of us don't have the time or the resources to go away. We have lives to lead and kids to raise. We need solutions that work, and that's exactly why I wrote this book. It's okay to make adjustments to fit your schedule if need be. But as I said earlier, I'm not suggesting that you intentionally blow it, but I am suggesting that you get back up and fight again if you fall.

Spiritual and physical health is not about perfection, but progress (I will remind you of this often). God uses failure to keep us humble. I've found that fasting is more about sowing than reaping, at least initially. Although there are incredible times of spiritual strength and devotion to the Lord, as well as high levels of energy, fasting can be very challenging, but the harvest will come when we sow according to God's Word.

Granted, there are times when breakthroughs come quickly, but more often than not, it takes time. *View fasting as planting seeds rather than consuming fruit.* But the fruit will come—God will never fail you; His Word is always true.

Be encouraged. We all struggle with something. *Use your weakness as a stepping stone rather than a stumbling block.* The Apostle Paul said, "When I am weak, then I am strong." He prayed three times for God to remove something from his life, but instead of removing it, God reminded him that His grace was (and is) sufficient. Your greatest weakness can also become a great catalyst toward a deeper relationship with God. What the enemy is using for evil God can use for good. Surrender everything to Him.

AVOID EXTREME FITNESS

As we begin, it's important to avoid extremes. In the health and fitness industry, there is something known as *orthorexia*. Although I don't agree with how some define *orthorexia*, it's viewed as an unhealthy focus on healthy food, or on having a perfect diet. Healthy living becomes an unhealthy obsession.[1] For example, I have heard of people who work out three times a day. This is not healthy or beneficial, and it can develop into a neurosis. I have also seen people become very upset at a waitress for accidentally placing cheese on their order. This type of behavior is not good.

I do, however, have concerns with the orthorexia label when it's used against health-conscious people without cause. We shouldn't be labeled with orthorexia simply because we want to live healthy and pass health on to our children. Childhood obesity is skyrocketing and we must do something. Lieutenant General Mark Hertling once spoke on this a decade ago under the title, *Obesity is a National Security Issue*.[2] Many young adults can't even pass basic military physical fitness exams, and many children are being diagnosed with diet-related diabetes. Parents, we must own this and change it.

To offset an unhealthy obsession, don't be so hard on yourself or others. Allow a treat now and then, enjoy food, and don't focus on having a perfect body. *A perfect ten is not our goal, but a healthy, God-honoring body is.* Eat to live; don't live to eat.

My wife and I try not to force healthy living on our kids, but we do influence and educate them. We want them to see the benefits and make their own choices as they get older. This is a hard balance to find, but it can be done if we make health a lifestyle and not an obsession.

For those who live in places that don't provide nutritious food, such as homes where parents aren't health-conscious or in hospital facilities that don't provide healthy options, God sees your heart. Focus on Him. You can only do what you can only do.

AVOID EXTREME FASTING

There's also a danger in taking fasting to the extreme. Like most things, it can be misapplied and misused. If you find yourself obsessed with performance, appearance, competition, and striving to fast, it may be best to take a break for a season.

After a few years of fasting before I would preach, I realized that it had become a routine that I no longer enjoyed. So I took a break. I thought that the break would have a negative effect on my preaching, but I was pleasantly surprised that it did not. After a year's break from fasting, I felt the need to start fasting again. It resulted in three forceful messages that reached over a million people on social media during the COVID lockdown in 2020. The links are in the footnote.[3]

POWERFUL FASTING TESTIMONY–*FAST, FOCUS, FAITH*

A friend of mine sent this to me while I was working on this book: "I personally had no self-control and I didn't see the benefits of an intentional fast. In 2019, I wrote in my notebook a text message from Diane Idleman that said, *"Try to abstain from anything that brings you pleasure or sustenance, but only do it with a purposeful intent or your fast will have no meaning and no power."*

"Something that really touched me was when I learned one of our youth completed a lengthy fast over the summer and, yet I couldn't commit for one week. I realized then that I had no control."

"In October 2020, I completed a thirty-day water/broth fast. Then I went to one meal a day for thirty days. It's been personal and POWERFUL! I have been purposeful and humble, and for the first time in my sixty years of life, I realize that I do have control . . . my relationship with the Lord has meaning like never before."

"It took about a full week to feel as though I wasn't punishing myself or thinking about it constantly. I felt hungry at about 3 or 4 p.m. each day, but I spoke to the Lord constantly. I found myself saying, 'I don't need food Lord, it will distract me. I need You'. When my stomach felt empty, it was like an alarm going off bringing me back to my focus. It's been a new mindset for me."

"Hunger pangs have a new meaning. It doesn't mean, 'Fill yourself with food', it means, 'There is business to take care of with God'. There is a lot of work to be done, and also many burdens and sorrows I've given to God these last few months. I could go on, but let me just say that, at first, you may feel weak, but give it time and you will have strength and faith that is unexplainable. People may think they are going to miss something by sacrificing a meal; when in fact you will be gaining spiritual food that you can't afford to miss. God is not done with me yet, I have much to do. FAST... FOCUS... FAITH."

WHY FORTY AND WHY FASTING?

"Fasting . . . when exercised with a pure heart and a right motive, may provide us with a key to unlock doors where other keys have failed" (Arthur Wallis).[1]

The number forty appears many times in the Bible—from forty-day fasts to forty days before judgment on Nineveh, and from forty days of Goliath taunting Israel to forty days to flood the earth. Jesus even stayed on earth for forty days after His resurrection. It appears that the number forty is significant.

Although it's been said that it takes twenty-one days to form a good habit, it often takes more time to deeply instill that habit and to remove bad habits. Those in addiction recovery, for example, are often still vulnerable after just a few weeks when *Post-acute Withdrawal Syndrome* kicks in.[2] Those fighting a food, sugar, or caffeine addiction also need more than just a few weeks to overcome it.

Forty days prepares the mind and the body both spiritually and physically. It provides sufficient time for serious change to take place. However, I don't recommend lengthy fasts for most people. My advice for the beginner would be to work up to a 24 or 36 hour fast on the weekends while maintaining a very healthy (primarily plant-based diet). There are many different options at your disposal that can lead to success (more on this later).

In some cases, it can take a month to start feeling better and for the body to adapt to a new way of living. Physically speaking, it takes time for taste buds to transition over to new food choices. Healthy, God-given foods that were once detested can taste good again. And spiritually speaking, it also takes time to renew the mind and build intimacy with God.

DISSECTING THE CAUSE OF DISEASE

For those choosing not to fast, consider using forty days to increase overall health. Turn off the media, go on walks, get to bed early, remove stimulants, and eat healthy. Researchers are finding that health is more *metabolic* than *genetic*. In other words, what we eat plays a significant role in either overcoming disease or fueling it. Fasting experts suggest that fasting can add a decade or two to one's life.

Although we may be pre-disposed to certain diseases, our lifestyle and food choices often determine the outcome more than our genes. Epigenetics (how our genes respond) and the study of the microbiome (gut bacteria) are both discovering that certain foods activate certain messengers in our RNA that affect our DNA in positive or negative ways.

For instance, if a certain type of cancer runs in your family—"it's in your genes," they say. But that doesn't necessarily mean you have to suffer with it. In many cases, consuming dead food signals certain rogue cells to divide in an unhealthy manner while spreading to other parts of the body (cancer is forming). But consuming living plant food places cancer-fighting phytochemicals as well as vitamins, minerals, and enzymes directly into the body. This doesn't mean that those who eat plants (think legumes, greens, and potatoes) will never get sick, but it does greatly increase the odds of maintaining health.

Dr. Joel Fuhrman notes that "factors such as hormones, adequacy of blood supply, and various unknown influences can affect cancer growth."[3] Fasting is not a cure-all, it simply provides an atmosphere in which healing can take place as the body speeds up the process of cleansing and renewing.

STARVE THE FUEL SOURCE

Changing our lifestyle is hard at first, but over forty days a pattern will develop. But let's not forget the most important part of the forty-day reset: *To renew the mind* (cf. Romans 12:2). For this reason, the daily reflections focus more on spiritual than physical health. We must be vigilant in our pursuit of God that begins in the mind.[4]

Here is where fasting comes into play: *Fasting can break down strongholds, starve the fuel source of sin, and renew the mind.* For example, in regard to overcoming addiction, health expert, Herbert Shelton, wrote, "Nothing enables the alcoholic, the drug fiend, and the tobacco addict to overcome his desire for his accustomed poison and to return to a state of good health, as does fasting."[5] This could also be said about those addicted to food. But be prepared, it's a fight! The flesh always wants to negotiate: "Can't we meet in the middle? Don't remove food—that's too extreme!" There are times, however, when God instantly delivers us from addiction, but often, we must starve our cravings instead of feeding them. *We strengthen what we feed.*

In regard to renewing the mind, fasting allows us to concentrate our thoughts toward God throughout the entire day—exchanging meal time for prayer time. Fasting also deprives the flesh of its appetites as we pray and seek God's will and mercy. We are saying, "The flesh got me into this predicament, now it's time to seek God's mercy and humble myself before Him."

Imagine heading to lunch in a crowded mall. Just before leaving, you notice that your three-year-old has disappeared—panic sets in! You must find your child at any cost. Are you going to eat first? Not a chance. The passion to find your child is far greater than the desire to eat. That's exactly what fasting is: *The desire to seek God is greater than the desire to eat.*

FIGHTING FOR REST

Rest means to be calm, wait patiently, lay down, put aside, and cease from activity. "Rest is a blessing which properly belongs to the people of God" (Charles Spurgeon).[6] Although most of us cannot completely shut down for forty days, we can renew our focus and restore energy as well as enthusiasm during this time. Renewed focus on rest often has a lasting impact.

Parents, I know it's hard, but we should model rest to our children by slowing down. Kids today are being raised in a very unhealthy and fast-paced world. There is little time for God as we hurry to our next destination, then run across town to drop them off somewhere for something, then hurry back home to eat dinner in separate rooms glued to computer screens until they pass out from sheer exhaustion. Something must change! I know that *fighting for rest* sounds like an oxymoron, but is something we must do.

Husbands and wives you may need to watch the kids now and then while allowing your spouse to spend time with God. You will need to fight for quiet moments as well. Today, Bible reading and prayer are called fanatical while working twelve hours a day is called success. We build our careers and neglect our marriage. Corporate executives are praised and family men frowned upon. Something must change. Dads, lead the way. We are watchmen, not showmen![7]

WE WAIT FOR WHAT WE VALUE

Fortunately, rest prevents burnout while providing clarity and peace. When the competing voice of busyness is briefly silenced, we hear more clearly from God. The Sabbath was designed for this reason: *To encourage less work and more time with God.* We would do well to follow that same model. Even if you can't take time off per se, turn your phone off and turn your attention toward God. Find a quiet place each day, even if it is for a short time. Rest your mind by reading a good book instead of looking at social media, especially before bed and upon arising. Trust me, we can find many ways to rest if we really want to.

One benefit of fasting is that you'll have extra time. Use this precious time to rest, pray, and seek God rather than being bored, restless, and moody. Remember Isaiah's words from earlier, that those who wait for and rest in the Lord will renew their strength (40:30-31). Waiting on the Lord shows how much we value hearing from Him. *We wait for what we value.* Like a desert that waits for the rain or a bride waiting for her groom, our longing must be for God. Prioritize times in your day to pray and build intimacy with Him . . . it won't happen on its own.[8]

HELP! I DON'T KNOW HOW TO PRAY?

Remember that prayer is based on having a genuine relationship with God. Because millions of people pray to *a god* every day, but not to the true God as identified in Scripture, you must begin here. Repentance and faith in Christ is the key that opens the prayer door.

Begin with a peaceful heart, an uninterrupted hour, and a quiet place. Simply reflect on the day behind and the day ahead. Ask for forgiveness if warranted and strength for the day. Ask God to speak to you through His Word. He isn't concerned with eloquence, but sincerity. Talk to Him like you would another person. Share your frustrations and fears as well as your hopes and joys.

I also listen to worship music for an hour in the morning. It takes a few minutes to eventually calm my mind and focus on God. This is one reason why I gave up coffee. I became too antsy, distracted, and irritable. I also try to not look at texts or emails for a few hours, and definitely not the news. My attention is on hearing from God.

I then read the Bible for an hour or so. While reading, I note scriptures that jump out and words to look up later in the Greek and Hebrew dictionaries. Granted, you may only have twenty minutes rather than two hours, and the Bible may seem confusing at first; that's okay—begin where you can. My podcast, *Why is the Bible So Confusing? What About All the Inconsistencies?* will help you in this area (see footnote).[9]

Like any other relationship, time together with God in prayer will lead to a deeper relationship. Don't be nervous—step out in faith and trust that God will speak to you.[10]

FASTING APPLIES PRESSURE TO THE SPIRITUAL REALM

Two opposing wills cannot successfully live in the same body—our self-will and God's will cannot co-exist in harmony.

With fast-food restaurants and convenience stores on every corner, it's no surprise that many people are in serious bondage to food and drink, and ironically, bondage in one area often opens the door for strongholds in other areas. *If abundance is the problem then abstinence via fasting is the solution.*

I'm startled at how many Christians don't practice fasting even though it's taught many times in the Bible. Jesus said that when He is taken away that His disciples would fast (cf. Matthew 9:15). The excuses range from "It's not for us today," and the infamous, "I'm just not convicted about fasting," to my personal favorite, "fasting is legalistic." Leonard Ravenhill was famous for saying, "The things in the Bible that we don't like we call legalism," and that definitely applies to excuses about fasting. The bottom line is that many people don't want to impeach King Stomach.[1]

THE POWER OF FASTING

The following section from my book, *Feasting and Fasting*, sheds more light on this important topic from a spiritual perspective:

In Matthew 17:21, Jesus said that a certain evil spirit does not go out of a person except by prayer and fasting. Some manuscripts disagree on whether this verse should be included or not, but the principle is found throughout Scripture: *Fasting applies pressure to the spiritual realm.* Arthur Wallis notes, "Often, pressure has to be maintained before there is a breakthrough in heavenly warfare."[2] It appears that some demonic activity is not released until pressure is applied through prayer and fasting.

The weapons we use to fight Satan are not physical; they are spiritual. The weapons should match the warfare! Satan cannot be eliminated with an AR-15, but we *can* fast and pray. Those two high-caliber spiritual bullets do substantial damage. Open the Word, pray, meditate, and worship for the fatal blow: "'Not by might nor by power, but by My Spirit,' says the Lord of hosts" (Zech. 4:6).

Two opposing wills cannot successfully live in the same body—our self-will and God's will cannot co-exist in harmony. We can't defeat what we feed. God's Word states, "For all that is in the world—the lust of the flesh, the lust of the eyes, and the pride of life—is not of the Father but is of the world" (1 John 2:16). Society says, "Be yourself! Embrace your longings! Feed your desires!" However, we know that gluttony and indulging the flesh never lead to spiritual victory, or any victory for that matter.

Some strongholds hang on piece by piece. We must "resist the devil" and he will eventually flee (James 4:7). *Fasting disciplines the body, prayer and worship bind the enemy, and the Word provides wisdom.* Fasting ignites a hunger for God and provides more time to seek Him.

Obviously, people have overcome challenges without fasting, but fasting adds extra strength, especially when overcoming addictions. Sadly, although one addiction may end, others can continue. The alcoholic switches to caffeine, the nicotine addict switches to sugar, and the opioid user switches to food. It's a never-ending cycle, but fasting can break the cycle. However, fasting is not a cure-all; it's a spiritual discipline designed to aid in victory.

TEN SPIRITUAL BENEFITS OF FASTING.

1. Fasting often leads to awakening, renewal, and spiritual restoration.
2. Fasting is a powerful prayer of intercession.
3. Fasting intensifies prayer.
4. Fasting removes pride and ushers in humility.
5. Fasting increases faith.
6. Fasting aids in overcoming obstacles.
7. Fasting crucifies the flesh and breaks bad habits.
8. Fasting and anointing go hand-in-hand.
9. Fasting helps to overcome unbelief.
10. Fasting opens doors that might not otherwise open.[3]

TEN PHYSICAL BENEFITS OF FASTING

Disease is often a problem of toxicity created by what we consume, ingest, and breathe—fasting is the detox solution. Granted, spiritual health and wholeness are the goals when fasting, but the physical benefits are worthwhile. Dr. J. H. Tilden once noted, "After fifty-five years of sojourning in the wilderness of medical therapeutics, I am forced to declare . . . that fasting is the only reliable, specific, therapeutic eliminant known to man."[4]

1. Fasting lowers blood pressure significantly as well as cleanses the blood.
2. Fasting is the best way to reduce weight and maintain a healthy weight.
3. Fasting rejuvenates the body, including the promotion of new stem cells and telomeres. Telomeres aid in rejuvenation and vitality. "Telomeres are made of repetitive sequences of non-coding DNA that protect the chromosome from damage. Each time a cell divides, the telomeres become shorter. Eventually, the telomeres become so short that the cell can no longer divide."[5] Fasting can delay this process.
4. Fasting helps to eliminate inflammation while allowing major organs such as the kidney, liver, digestive tract, and heart to rest and repair.
5. Fasting helps to prevent cardiovascular disease and aids in the removal of atherosclerosis (hardening of the arteries) by breaking it down.[6]
6. Fasting leads to mental clarity and brain health.
7. Fasting can shrink certain tumors. When the body is low on fuel, it will consume the non-functional cells as autophagy runs its course.
8. Fasting is very effective in offsetting diabetes and other health-related diseases.
9. Fasting helps with depression and anxiety.
10. Fasting has been shown to help with rheumatoid arthritis, gout, eczema, and psoriasis.

In short, since most diseases are fueled by what we consume, removing the fuel source allows the body to rebuild, cleanse, and repair.

BE ON GUARD IN THESE TWO AREAS

A key component of peace and rest, from a physical standpoint, is our diet. What you consume may be consuming you.

Most restlessness comes from two primary sources—*mental and physical stress.* Thoughts determine our level of peace and rest. A constant mental diet of negative news, mesmerizing media, and ungodly, dark entertainment will surely lead to fear and frustration. This is exactly why Romans 12:2 declares, "Do not be conformed to this world, but be transformed by the renewing of your mind, that you may prove what is that good and acceptable and perfect will of God."

What you read, watch, and listen to is either fostering peace or fueling fear. Take steps now and remove things that are hurting mental and spiritual health. Procrastination is the great enemy of accomplishment. Even if you can't rest as often as you'd like, you can be at peace if your mind is fixed on the things of God.

Another key component of peace and rest, from a physical standpoint, is our diet. Yes, you heard me correctly: *what you consume may be consuming you.* Did you know that God-given food brings life to the body, and dead food depletes it? A poor diet, followed by inactivity and weight gain, forces us to run on only two cylinders as opposed to all eight. It hurts our efficiency and productivity as well as our mental capacity. Ironically, one of the benefits of fasting is mental *clarity*. Granted, as stated earlier, there are those who, through no fault of their own, have a debilitating illness. I'm assuming the reader understands that I'm talking to those who *can* make changes.

Certain foods raise the levels of serotonin in the brain. This neurotransmitter is responsible for feelings of peace, wellness, and calmness. Sadly, most people consume dead food that depletes instead of food that restores. Add the damaging effects of massive sugar consumption to a poor diet, high stress, and a lack of sleep, and it's no surprise why health-related illnesses (physical and mental) have reached epidemic levels.

Most of our bodies are in a very toxic state because we are consuming dead food and dangerous stimulants, and we rarely fast. When we get sick, we struggle to heal. It's disheartening when people take a pill or a shot to offset disease instead of using the God-given method of fasting and consuming healthy food.

TERRORISTS WITHIN OUR BODY

Here is an excerpt from my book on fasting that explains how unhealthy choices are like terrorists within the body:

1. Unhealthy food consists of growth hormones, antibiotics, drug residue, pathogens, biotoxins, chemicals, and carcinogens. These things are like terrorists to the body.
2. If high levels of sugar, such as high fructose corn syrup,

dextrose, maltose, rice syrup, sucrose, and dozens more, are added to the terrorism team, the strength of the enemy grows.[1]
3. If we add massive amounts of refined vegetable oils to the terrorism team, arteries and healthy cells become damaged due to inflammation.
4. Add the failure to fast to the equation and the enemy gains additional ground. Fasting invites *SEAL Team Six* to the battle. Among other things, fasting starves the fuel source of free radicals because most toxins are released during the digestion of food. Imagine what a bowl of junk cereal releases into your body compared to nothing being released when fasting. I believe that fasting slows aging for this very reason: *It minimizes toxins while allowing the body to cleanse and rebuild.*
5. Throw inactivity into the battle, and the terrorists gain even more strength. Our bodies were not designed to sit for long periods. Every pound of fat requires a few extra miles of blood vessels. That means more work for the body, especially the heart. Lose the excess and bring in more reinforcements.

Research the effects of stress on the body as well as how sleep affects health. If we combine all these factors, it's easy to see why disease has reached epidemic levels and has prevented genuine rest. Work on these areas for forty days, and you can change the course of the battle in your favor.

All of this, however, will not lead to *true* peace until you know the Prince of Peace and commit your life to Christ. Take this step today. There is no Plan B: "Come to me, all you that labor and are heavy laden, and I will give you rest. Take my yoke on you, and learn of me; for I am meek and lowly in heart: and you shall find rest to your souls" (Matthew 11:28-29). As Charles Spurgeon wisely said, "O you who feel your unworthiness this morning, who have been seeking salvation earnestly, and suffering the weight of sin, Jesus will freely give to you what you cannot earn or purchase."[2]

STIMULANTS—ROBBING PETER AND PLUNDERING PAUL

It's amazing how we make excuses to indulge in things that harm us. We love good news about bad habits.

I bet you didn't know that a major hindrance to health and rest is something that we use daily—*caffeine*. Caffeine plays a huge role in anxiety and restlessness. It often fuels angry temper tantrums and explosive outbursts, as well as irritability and a quick temper. No surprise here: *What's eating you may have to do with what you're eating, or drinking.*

Most people know that poor food choices affect *physical* health, but they fail to see the connection with *mental* health. Stimulants, poor food choices, and medication all play a role in mental instability. Even the *Diagnostic and Statistical Manual for Mental Disorders* lists caffeine-related disorders. Did you catch that? If we believe we can drink a high-powered stimulant (or take a depressant) day in and day out and not have it affect our rest and peace, we are gravely mistaken.[1] When we feed the body what it *needs*, rather than what it *wants*, everything works better.

Why would we consume caffeine (in coffee or strong tea) if we're trying to rest the heart and avoid harmful chemicals and pesticides during a fast, or when we're trying to minimize stress? It makes no sense.

Caffeine may provide temporary relief, but you're robbing Peter and plundering Paul. There is no upside. You may say, "Shane, haven't you read articles about the benefits of coffee?" First, research who paid for the study. It was probably the coffee industry. Second, that's like telling an alcoholic to enjoy a glass of wine because of the antioxidant benefits (just eat grapes). Third, addiction is addiction no matter how it's excused. Fourth, constantly amping up the body comes with a price such as damage to the cardiovascular system.

I once saw a sign above a coffee pot in a doctor's office that said: "DON'T CONSUME BEFORE A STRESS TEST." Need I say more? Let's wake up; our health is on the line. It's amazing how we make excuses to indulge in things that harm us. Sadly, even when I share this information about stimulants, very few want to change. *As they say, "We love good news about bad habits."*

I know that many people don't *want* to hear this, but we *need* to hear it. If a person is gulping down coffee and stopping frequently for energy drinks, they'll never find rest. They may argue, "But I fall asleep just fine." That's because the body is exhausted and it crashes due to adrenal fatigue. Caffeine, along with alcohol and opiates, is why many people can't get a good night's sleep and wake up refreshed. We must seek to eliminate these hindrances if we truly want to experience rest and peace.

All of this begs the question, *"How many are suffering mentally and physically simply because of poor health choices—continuing the addiction rather than removing the cause of the problem?"* You may go through difficult withdrawals, but rest and peace are just around the corner.

If you begin a fast while drinking coffee, consider weaning off the first week by adding organic decaf and decreasing regular coffee by half each day until it's at zero. Even though you may be tired, this approach will ease withdrawals and help remove the addiction.

IF YOU FAIL, FALL FORWARD

"For all of life is like race, with ups and downs and all, and all you have to do to win is rise each time you fall."

Although I do believe that the best type of fast is to drink clean, pure water, there are other things that you can do such as drinking juice, eating healthy food, cutting out sugar, fasting intermittently, and so on (more on that later).

It's also great to take a break from the negative news and unproductive entertainment during this time, but fasting, in the truest sense of the word, is refraining from eating or drinking anything that delivers nutrients to your body. However, if a person can't fast (or fast perfectly), isn't it better for them to end the forty-day challenge twenty pounds lighter and feeling great even though they didn't fast or eat perfectly?

Isn't it better for a person to eat a handful of nuts during a fast if they feel terrible but need to coach their kids' sports team? Isn't it better for a person to overcome alcohol, nicotine, or pain meds even though they didn't do things perfectly? ABSOLUTELY!

When life throws a curveball, get back up to the plate and swing again.

Caving in doesn't necessarily take you all the way back to the starting line, and eating a bad meal doesn't reverse all of your hard work. Yes, most of the time, it's best to fight through the detox process and experience the full benefits of fasting and/or clean eating, but we also need encouragement to continue moving forward despite setbacks. *Viewing detox symptoms as healing pains will help you push through.*

DON'T LISTEN TO THE ARMCHAIR QUARTERBACKS

As I follow fasting forums on social media, I'm amazed at how many arrogant arm-chair quarterbacks stand on the sidelines critiquing those who don't follow their exact protocol. Instead of encouraging people, they say things like, "If you put lemon juice in your water, drink herbal tea, and chew gum with xylitol, you're not really fasting. You blew it. Start over!" GIVE ME A BREAK!

Granted, consuming minimal amounts of nutrients can temporarily disengage cleansing, but nit-picking and critiquing others is not helpful. Don't let the Negative-Nellies, Judgemental-Jerrys, or the Critical-Cathys sidetrack you; most of them don't fast perfectly themselves. Don't quit if you slip and lose your footing. Get back up!

Hardcore fasting advocates may not agree, but that's okay. They aren't in your shoes. Your forty-day reset should be practical as well as powerful. Recall what I said earlier: We need encouragement and grace to push through.

HUMILITY THROUGH FAILURE

As a perfectionist (or at least I try to be), from reading this manuscript over twenty times looking for the perfect words, to having my desk spotless and clean, God has taught me a great deal through failure in key areas of my life, and one such area is fasting. When I do things in my own strength and try to be *perfect*, I fall flat on my face. It's clear that I need His grace and mercy on a daily basis. God often uses failure to keep us humble.

Even with my fasting experience mentioned later in this book, I didn't do things perfectly. I went days with just water, then I ate a little if I had to do a project, take a trip, or handle an important issue. Instead of beating myself up because I missed perfection (or what is perceived as perfection), I *failed forward* and kept going, and so should you. As a famous poem declares: "For all of life is like race, with ups and downs and all, and all you have to do to win is rise each time you fall."[1]

Regardless of whether you're on your 100th diet attempt or can't seem to make health a lifestyle, get back up and fight again. "Success is not final, failure is not fatal: it is the courage to continue that counts" (Winston Churchill). And Henry Ford reminds us, "When everything seems to be going against you, remember that an airplane takes off against the wind, not with it." *Fail forward.*

WHAT TYPE OF FAST SHOULD I DO?

For those who can't fast for a variety of reasons, we can all make important changes that will change the course of our lives and the lives of our children.

Many of the suggestions in this chapter are not fasting protocols; they are healthy eating programs. There are a lot of creative ideas, but the definition of fasting is to abstain from any regular source of strength and nourishment, food and liquid.

Fasting is not something that we should fear. *We should fear excessive fat, but not fasting.* The word *fasting* in the Bible means to abstain from all forms of nutrients and drink water. Granted, not everyone can take time off to fast, and some people shouldn't fast, but others can fast and maintain their schedule. For instance, J. Harold Smith, in his book *Fast Your Way to Health*, stated that he was able to do a twenty-eight day fast consuming just water while maintaining his busy schedule.[1]

Throughout the book, I use the words *water fasting* to describe fasting while drinking water, rather than meaning fasting *from* water. (I did a modified version of this type of fast in the chapter about my fasting experience.) In the Bible, Daniel was the exception. He avoided all appealing food. One reason the Daniel approach was (and still is) so powerful, is because the body consumes only God-given food. I call it the *Daniel Healthy Eating Plan* instead of a fast.

Although there isn't a one-size-fits-all approach, I can offer a few suggestions. Before beginning, ask God for direction and confirmation. For many, the best solution is to simply step out in faith. God gave us wisdom (through His Word) and faith (in His Son) to navigate our lives.

FASTING WHILE CONSUMING JUST WATER

As I discussed in the section, *Fasting Applies Pressure to the Spiritual Realm*, the primary focus of a fast should be for spiritual reasons, but we should also take care of our incredible body that God gifted us.

Those fasting to improve physical health should allow their body to determine the length. The old adage, "Let nature dictate the length of the fast," is very true. If the fast ends too soon, the faster will miss many of the wonderful healing benefits. Therefore, unless God leads you otherwise, it may be wise not to start a fast using water when you're approaching a busy period of life, or when you need to spend time with others biking, camping, and so on. During a busy season, consider light juicing and healthy eating in preparation for a fast. Then, when the time is right, step out in faith as Jesus instructs in Matthew 6:16—"When you fast."

From my experience, going into a fast with a clean diet while fasting intermittently for a few weeks prior, makes a world of difference. Water fasting isn't nearly as challenging when the body is ready for it.

During a water fast, many biological changes take place that require weeks to fully exhaust. Many of the detox symptoms will eventually disappear when the body has finished the process of cleansing. I've witnessed eyesight improving, tumors shrinking, arthritis healing, addictions being broken, and many other things improving during a lengthy fast (e.g., three to six weeks is not uncommon). In most cases, as long as the faster is not in poor health and/or has little fat reserves, the longer the fast the better.

Due to excessive amounts of fat stored in our bodies, most people can fast for a significant amount of time. Technically speaking, being thirty pounds overweight with approximately 105,000 stored calories means that one could fast for approximately fifty days on those energy reserves. Vitamin and mineral reserves, along with other factors, would also play a role in determining the length.

In 1973, a 27-year-old man water-fasted for 382 days under the supervision of the Scotland University. His weight dropped from 456 lbs. to 180 lbs. and he was able to maintain a healthy weight when eating resumed.[2] But again, it's wise to seek medical advice when fasting long-term. There are those who shouldn't do lengthy fasts such as those on medication or those with borderline kidney failure and things of that nature.

Some recommend drinking distilled water when fasting. Because distilled water contains no minerals, the thought process is that the body will pull from its own mineral storage tanks, thus allowing deeper autophagy to take place. I assume, however, that most people in biblical times drank mineral-rich water since minerals come from the water interacting with the soil. But, at other times, people drank rainwater that contained no trace minerals. I don't have a strong view on this because a lot depends on the length of the fast, the health of the faster, and the amount of reserves that they have. Personally, I don't drink distilled water very often. I choose clean water obtained through reverse osmosis.

THE FASTING MIMICKING DIET

For those who cannot fast, some suggest a fasting mimicking diet for five days followed by healthy eating for two days. During a fasting mimicking diet, around 500-800 calories are consumed each day consisting of foods low in protein and carbohydrates, but high in healthy fat. Dr. Valter Longo, *Director of the Longevity Institute at USC*, has good information on this type of protocol. In my case, this type of program is often harder than water fasting because the constant desire to eat is always gnawing at me, but for others, it's a good place to start.

FASTING INTERMITTENTLY

Another alternative to fasting is something known as *intermittent fasting*, or IF. It's very popular because it provides some of the basic benefits of fasting without really fasting. Granted, the benefits are not nearly as beneficial as water fasting, but it has helped many people. When I eat intermittently, I consume only water for sixteen to twenty hours, then I consume healthy meals in a small window. An example would be grilled organic chicken on a huge, very colorful salad with homemade dressing and a baked potato followed by a large organic smoothie later in the evening.

Under this heading, *One Meal a Day (OMAD)* is also popular. The famous prayer warrior, Rees Howells, did this for months as he prayed for the end of WWII. The key for both intermittent fasting and OMAD is not to overindulge (gluttony) when you do eat.

THOUGHTS ON JUICING

Juicing continually supplies the body with nutrients, but we won't receive the same type of deep cleaning as with water only because our body uses the juice for fuel rather than allowing autophagy and ketosis to take place. So it really depends on what your goals are. Autophagy is when the body uses diseased and old tissues and cells for fuel, and ketosis is when our body begins using fat for fuel. Both are God-given processes that begin a few days into a water fast to renew and restore the body. As with IF, the benefits are not nearly as beneficial as water fasting, but juicing has helped many people.

Juicing keeps the pancreas, liver, digestive tract, and other organs very active. This defeats the purpose of fasting to rest the body. One may lose weight drinking juice because of caloric restriction, and autophagy will take place to some degree during sleep (our body is always removing, adding, and renewing), but overall, it's not the best way to reap the full benefits of fasting unless one's health prevents fasting. For example, juicing may be the best option and a good first step for those whose health has deteriorated and for those on medication.

I don't think that we were created to consume the fruit of three oranges, four apples, and five broccoli sticks all in one sitting. The pulp is exceptionally good for the body and should be consumed with the juice when we eat the entire piece of produce. The pulp also helps regulate blood sugar levels by slowing down the absorption of the juice.

Juicing can also place harmful chemicals into your body if the fruits and vegetables are sprayed with chemicals—even organic food isn't always clean. However, not everyone can fast, or they may feel overwhelmed at the thought. In this case, juicing with organic produce is a good step forward and will prepare the body for future fasts. Start where you can. Small steps in the right direction will pay off.

WHAT IS DRY FASTING

Dry fasting occurs when nothing is consumed, not even water. Since our skin can absorb moisture, hard-core advocates don't let water touch their body whether through bathing or swimming. Personally, I'm not a fan of dry fasting even though I have heard of success stories. The thought is that it speeds up autophagy and fat loss because more fat cells are being utilized for hydration. Please use wisdom here; it can severely dehydrate the body. Even though I sometimes go ten hours with no water, say from 7 pm to 5 am, my advice is to drink when thirst demands it because hydration is very important when it comes to utilizing and transporting stored minerals.

REMAINING ACTIVE DURING A FAST

Long-term water fasting, while remaining active, can slow healing and should be avoided. The detoxifying benefits of fasting are hindered when autophagy can't run its course. Granted, our body is always breaking down cells and repairing, but rest kicks healing into high gear. Activity, such as strenuous exercise, breaks down muscle and converts it to glucose to fuel the immediate need. This is known as *gluconeogenesis*. Those who feel led to fast for health reasons should consider resting often to receive the highest benefit.

In the Bible, Jesus was in the wilderness and Moses was on a mountain for forty days while fasting. I'm assuming a lot of rest occurred. Elijah, on the other hand, walked a great distance in forty days on the strength of the food he ate weeks prior. God sustained him. That's the key: Let God guide you, use wisdom, seek godly counsel, and obey His Word: "The humble He teaches His way" (Psalm 25:9). Fasting is a step of humility that God honors as long as our heart is right.

For those who will remain active, following something like the *fasting mimicking diet* or *intermittent fasting* may be wise, or maybe consuming one large, healthy meal on activity days would be best. It's actually easier for me to work out after going sixteen hours without food. The key is to not overindulge when you finally do eat (you're still fasting to some degree).

For those who want to remain active, I've found that the best plan is to exercise daily. Aim for twenty to forty minutes of cardiovascular training each day followed by twenty minutes of resistance training while taking a day off each week. This consistent pattern leads to a consistent workout routine.

WHO SHOULDN'T FAST?

As stated before, those taking medication and other drugs should seek advice from their physician. For example, those taking high blood pressure medication while fasting must be careful because fasting substantially lowers blood pressure. If medication is combined with fasting, blood pressure may drop too low. Fasting also affects insulin. For those taking insulin while fasting, make sure your physician is aware. Fasting, when done correctly, has helped many people with type II diabetes lose weight and become medication-free.[3]

Another example of being careful with medication would be when diabetics use Metformin. Metformin prevents gluconeogenesis from taking place in the liver, but the body needs gluconeogenesis to take place during a fast. Gluconeogenesis is when the liver produces new glucose to fuel the body by breaking down protein or fat. The word literally means making glucose out of nothing: *gluco* for glucose, *neo* for new, and *genesis* for creation. Problems arise when a person needs the liver to produce glycogen when fasting, but then takes medication that prevents it from happening. Not good.

PREGNANT WOMEN

Women who are pregnant or who are nursing should avoid fasting because the baby needs key nutrients. Moms, this is the time to remove everything from caffeine to alcohol from your diet and eat clean, God-given food. The baby's health depends on it.

TOO THIN TO FAST

Those who are *very* thin and unhealthy should not attempt a long fast. Instead, try to build strength and increase health by eating whole, organic food. However, thin people, who have some fat reserves, have benefited greatly from fasting. They often gain the needed weight after the fast is over. The fast seems to *reset* the metabolism. It may also be wise for those struggling with eating disorders such as bulimia and anorexia to avoid fasting. "People who have anorexia severely reduce their food intake to lose weight. People who have bulimia eat an excessive amount of food in a short period of time, then purge or use other methods to prevent weight gain" (*Healthline.com*)[4]

Eating disorders are debilitating and affect more people than we realize, largely because of Hollywood's influence on appearance. As with all struggles, take it to God in prayer. Renew your mind through His Word and let the Holy Spirit guide you, not Hollywood. I also provided a helpful resource in the footnote.[5]

ELECTROLYTES AND WATER

Complications can also arise via electrolyte imbalances during long-term fasting. Drinking too much water can flush out electrolytes too quickly, while drinking too little water can lead to dehydration. Drink water based on thirst, and ask your physician about trace mineral supplements if need be. However, many fasting experts testify that the body has plenty of vitamin and mineral storage tanks. If you embark on a lengthy fast, have your physician monitor important things such as potassium and magnesium.

In my opinion, (although there may be exceptions), I wouldn't take supplements, herbs, or detox formulas when fasting. They often disturb the complicated balances of things in your body. For example, I've known people who used cleansing teas that contain such things as senna leaf and licorice. These ingredients triggered heart palpitations for these individuals for most of the day.

CONTROLLING THE REFEEDING MONSTER

We must use wisdom and caution in the area of refeeding. After a fairly long fast, it's important to properly refeed every few hours using light foods such as fruit, juice, or bone broth. Some may need to do this for a week depending on the length of the fast. If one starts eating large meals, or the wrong type of food right away, it can harm their body and may lead to complications including severe abdominal pain. To be forewarned is to be forearmed.

Here is an excerpt from a book on fasting:

> One gentleman that I worked with some years ago was doing great; he had reached day 21 of water fasting and had lost more than 30 pounds. But he did not do the house cleanup as I suggested. One afternoon, while he was navigating a tough wave of hunger, he opened the cupboard and found two boxes of corn and bran muffins, smiling and fervently calling his name. "Charles! Charles! Come to us, Charles!" He was vulnerable and, in spite of the amazing progress he had made, he opened the boxes and ate all 9 muffins. He called me in tears, feeling defeated and demoralized, not to mention that he fell ill; breaking a long fast inappropriately is very dangerous and could result in serious injury and even death. He had to go to the hospital and have his stomach pumped because the digestive system had been hibernating and could not handle the sudden intake of food. That incident could have been avoided if only Charles had been willing to follow some simple instructions. And I confess that the same thing happened to me when I first started fasting.[6]

The same amount of self-control is needed when ending the fast as was needed when the fast began. Please take this point seriously. I've eaten too much a few times and definitely paid the price. When eating is resumed, it's wise to plan ahead by laying out small meals for a few days. You may even consider going somewhere that doesn't have a full pantry and a packed refrigerator.

Once refeeding resumes, the body instinctively wants more and more food to refuel the storage tanks. It's very hard not to overindulge, and consuming a lot of food at once can disturb electrolyte levels which can lead to heart palpitations and feelings of depression and anxiety.[7] This is exactly what happened to me during a long fast (read about it in the chapter titled, *A Must Read Fasting Experience*).

Please make sure to research refeeding if you go longer than three days. Most experts recommend breaking a fast with light organic juice and possibly a few slices of an orange every few hours. Then slowly work in bone broth and steamed vegetables over the next few days (depending on how long the fast was). In my opinion, we need to be very careful in regard to carbohydrates at this stage. Overconsumption can increase inflammation and promote fat storage.[8]

Additionally, I wish it wasn't the case, but don't expect to feel really good during refeeding. When food is reintroduced, many biological changes take place in the body that can lead to aches and pains as well as feelings of being bloated along with increased inflammation. But the cleaner the diet the better you feel during refeeding.

After a long water fast, it's wise not to fast again for a significant amount of time in order for nutritional reserves to build up. For example, if you fast for three weeks using water only, it may be wise to wait a few months before fasting again. *The longer the fast, the longer the waiting period.*

As a final point, it's my understanding that fasting slows down the body's metabolism. Care must also be taken after the refeeding period to allow the metabolism to resume normal activity. This can take up to a month. Don't let discipline and self-control plummet when the fast ends. You will still need their help, especially if you don't want to return to your old ways.

FOR THOSE WHO CAN'T FAST

As you can see, it's very important to educate yourself before fasting.[9] For those who can't fast for a variety of reasons, remember that we all can make important changes that will change the course of our lives. Removing destructive influences from your life while eliminating unhealthy foods will benefit you greatly. For example, Daniel only ate healthy plant-based food and was greatly blessed by God.

What's stopping you? Remember, if it doesn't cost you anything, it may not mean anything. Like David, we should say, *I will not give God that which cost me nothing* (see 2 Samuel 24:24). Whatever the fast, it should involve denying the body something it craves. God sees your heart. Focus on Him, not on perfection.

THE HARDEST PART OF A FAST

What you eat will determine the course of your health more than the fast itself. Fasting isn't a cure, it simply sets the stage. Your diet is the main actor.

For most people, the endurance test takes place at the beginning and at the end of the fast. The first few days can be the hardest and the refeeding phase can be very challenging when the hunger monster is re-awakened. For this reason, I often include the re-feeding phase into the length of my fast. For example, if you fast for ten days using water, consider putting fourteen days on your calendar to include re-feeding. Too many of us can't wait to end the fast so we can indulge in everything that we missed. Although the main part may be over, you still need to be very careful when reintroducing food.

The diet following a fast should consist primarily of whole foods from plants. *What you eat after the fast will determine the course of your health far more than the fast itself.* I hope you caught that

—read that last sentence again. Lifestyle changes are the key to long-term success. Fasting isn't a cure, it simply provides the right environment for change to occur. Diet is the main player in the health game.

For others, the hardest part of a fast involves withdrawing from nicotine, caffeine, alcohol, sugar, processed foods, medication, and so on. We often say, "Fasting is killing me; it's too hard," and we give up and blame the fast. Instead, blame a poor diet and wean yourself off of destructive habits, then try fasting.

WHAT IF I BECOME SICK WHILE FASTING?

Fasting is challenging because of how we *feel*. Not only is the body switching to ketones as its fuel source during the first few days, it's also withdrawing from addictions and removing toxins. Unlike a cold or the flu where you have no other choice but to wait it out, with fasting, the discomfort can end by eating. It's truly a mental and physical challenge.

Experts are divided on whether you should push through when feeling sick or eat a small amount of food. There isn't an easier answer because it depends on what is making you sick. That's why it's wise to have a physician monitor progress. Being dehydrated and having a low potassium level, for example, is more of a concern than simply experiencing the keto-flu. "The so-called keto flu is a group of symptoms that may appear two to seven days after starting a ketogenic diet. Headache, foggy brain, fatigue, irritability, nausea, difficulty sleeping, and constipation are just some of the symptoms of this condition, which is not recognized by medicine" (Harvard Health).[1]

In my case, I press through as long as it is not intense and I don't have any scheduled commitments that would require sufficient energy. For example, if I feel sick and need energy to watch the kids, or to make an important event, I may choose to consume something liquid such as two cups of bone broth (thirty calories) or a scoop of healthy protein powder mixed with almond milk (175 calories).[2]

Although this may restore a minimal amount of energy, it's only temporary. Most who go this route, have to deal with sickness again until detox is complete. In essence, it's prolonging the inevitable. However, in certain circumstances, it may be wise to eat a little food. In the same way that a person weans off of medication, others may need to wean off of junk food. The liver and the kidneys can't always keep up with cleansing if too many toxins are released while fasting. This is especially true in the case of someone withdrawing from drugs. Consuming a small, nutrient-dense meal may help slow the effects of detox to a manageable level so the person can continue the fast. And they may have to do this a few times.

Die-hard fasting advocates may not agree with this approach, but that's okay. I'm not going to let a few calories sidetrack me, and neither should you. If a small amount of calories helps a person eventually accomplish their goal, is that a bad thing? Granted, I want to be clear here: *It's best to push through not feeling well if you can.* For example, if the full benefits of autophagy need to be experienced, then a doctor's supervision through the hard process may be best. But if you're extremely overweight, although drinking water only would be ideal, you may need to eat a few times to eventually reach your goal. I'd rather have a person hit their goal than quit: "A man full of hope will be full of action" (Thomas Brooks).[3] Others, however, may feel that God wants them to push through (I've done this many times). In all cases, use wisdom and do what you think is best. We all have different convictions, goals, and circumstances.

If you decide to consume a minimal amount of calories, be aware that it can spark hunger, hinder ketosis, and knock you out of autophagy for a short time. The more calories you consume, the more the healing process will be hindered. For example, thirty calories from bone broth won't hinder healing much at all (in my opinion), but consuming 400 calories from juice will definitely set you back. Drinking juice hinders ketosis and stops autophagy for many hours.

When possible, I recommend withdrawing from caffeine, sugar, processed food, alcohol, nicotine, and so on before beginning a fast. It makes the experience much more pleasant and sets you up for success once the fast is over. Other people, however, dive right in. I've known people who abused alcohol one day and began a lengthy fast the next day. They eventually felt good after the painful withdrawals subsided.[4] But again, make sure your physician is aware of your decision. Then use wisdom, step out in faith, rely on God, and get ready to experience the benefits of fasting.

THE MAINTENANCE CHALLENGE

Another big challenge is maintaining results and not reverting back to old eating patterns after the fast. There have been times when my joints felt great while fasting, but instead of eating healthy, I went back to chips and crackers, as well as meat and dairy when the fast was over. Even though the food was technically *organic,* it wasn't the best choice. Just because a label says organic (think organic Doritos or Oreos) doesn't mean that the food is beneficial, especially if it's man-made and contains things such as emulsifiers, refined oils, sugars, maltodextrin (a high glycemic carbohydrate), and so on.

The best choice, when possible, is organic God-given foods that have not been altered, enriched, or modified. For those wondering what exactly organic means, the *Rodale Institute* breaks it down: "A product with the USDA Certified Organic seal must be grown or produced with no synthetic herbicides, pesticides, or fertilizers—and that means no RoundUp and no glyphosate."

The article continues, "Organic not only bans synthetic herbicides like RoundUp—it prohibits the use of hundreds of chemical additives, preservatives, colorings, and more." Organic companies often use natural chemicals but not synthetic ones. See the full article in the footnote.[5]

During the maintenance phase, keep in mind that *healthy* isn't always *helpful*. A friend of mine, Dr. Daniel Pompa, recently commented about his visit to a leading health-food chain: *"I was stunned by how many harmful ingredients I found, even in supposedly 'paleo-friendly' or 'super-healthy' snacks!"*

One example he gave was how many food companies are allowed to slide in up to half a gram of trans fats per serving in their food and still claim their food is 'Trans Fat Free' (even though it isn't). Ninety-nine percent of beef sticks, for example, are preserved by coating them with citric acid and hydrogenated vegetable oil, which is trans fat. Yet, they can hide this by labeling it encapsulated citric acid. Pretty slick uh?

As another example, according to independent laboratory tests, certain brands of hummus were found to be contaminated with high levels of glyphosate (a weed-killing chemical linked to cancer).[6] Know what you're consuming.

MOTIVATION CHALLENGE

Motivation can be very challenging during a fast, so I found motivation by listening to the experience of others and reading helpful books (see the *Recommended Reading* list at the end of this book). In October 2020, my oldest daughter's example of drinking water for forty days motivated me greatly. A few weeks into her fast, I said, "Okay, that's long enough. Time to eat." But she said that she really felt led to continue because she was drawing closer to God. Having a background in health and fitness, I could tell that her body was responding in an amazing way, and I didn't want to stop her pursuit. Her electrolytes and mineral levels seemed fine. In regard to identifying low electrolytes, I look for muscle twitching, diarrhea, palpitations, extremely low energy, and so on. Although it's best to let the body release exactly what it needs and when, some people take trace mineral supplementation if need be. I was shocked when she completed the fast; it transformed her life.

She also lost over thirty-five pounds and kept half of it off even six months later. Although weight loss isn't the primary goal in a spiritual fast, it can be a very nice blessing. When we benefit spiritually we also often benefit physically.

THE SLEEP CHALLENGE

Many people have a hard time sleeping because fasting raises hormone levels that often cause restlessness. This is normal and should be expected. Stay up late if need be and read a positive and encouraging book.

To combat insomnia, some fasters use natural sleep aids such as valerian root or 5-HTP (5-hydroxytryptophan). Valerian root contains ingredients that promote sleep and relaxation; whereas

5-HTP is a by-product of the amino acid L-tryptophan which raises serotonin. I've used both of these separately from time to time. However, because they want the body in a pure state, most fasting experts discourage the use of sleeping aids, even natural ones. Additionally, the body doesn't need as much sleep when fasting.

Also keep in mind that your body will feel cold when fasting, especially at night, because heat isn't being produced from digestion. Changes to blood flow, along with a slower metabolism, often lead to feeling cold when fasting.

A QUICK NOTE ON WEIGHT LOSS/GAIN

Another challenge that many have is dealing with the weight that is gained back when the fast is over. Depending on your weight, it's not uncommon to lose two to four pounds a day at the beginning of the fast. The large amount of weight that is lost in the first few days is primarily from stored glycogen being depleted and the water it holds, along with waste in the digestive tract. This weight will come back when eating is resumed, but you can expect to lose about a half-pound of fat per day and keep it off if you maintain a healthy lifestyle after the fast.

For example, if a person loses twenty-eight pounds on a twenty-one-day fast, approximately ten of those pounds may be from fat. The rest comes from stored glycogen and tissue that is consumed during autophagy. A pound or two of muscle can be used as fuel as well depending on the fasters activity level as well as their genetic composition, growth hormone levels, etc. But I'd rather experience the incredible benefits of fasting and lose a little muscle (that can easily be regained), than hold on to a small amount of muscle and miss the benefits of fasting.

The weight that is gained back once eating is resumed initially comes from refueling the glycogen tanks. This gain is primarily water and stored carbohydrates, not fat. So if you want to lose thirty pounds, you may consider fasting until you've lost at least forty.

Many studies show that fat does not come back easily if a healthy diet is maintained. In many cases, the person continues to burn fat when the fast is over if they don't over-indulge in carbohydrates or calories. Fasting is a true reset as long as a healthy lifestyle follows it.

SHOULD WE KEEP OUR FAST PRIVATE?

For those who think that we should keep our fasts private, how did we know that Jesus and others fasted in the Bible? Because they told others. In Matthew 6:16, Jesus didn't say not to tell anyone, He said don't boast and brag (the opposite of humility); don't give the impression that you're fasting (showing off). If the heart is right, it's acceptable to share a fasting experience with others if God releases you to do so (there are times, however, to keep it private).

Sharing our experience can motivate and encourage others. Fasting changed my life and I simply want to share this great biblical truth with others. But be careful: it may be wise not to share what you're doing immediately with friends and family. Many think that fasting is weird, monastic, extreme, and so on. Their comments can knock you off track and discourage progress. I recall one such day in 2019 when I walked into the church ready to preach a message that God laid on my heart during a nine-day fast. One of the older members said something like, "You look too skinny. You need to eat." Sadly, this man needed to lose a lot of weight and was in poor health. My heart broke for him. Even though I was able to re-focus, I still remember his words.

BIBLICALLY SPEAKING, WHAT SHOULD I EAT?

Genetics load the gun, lifestyle pulls the trigger. The food you eat can be either the safest and most powerful form of medicine or the slowest form of poison.[1]

There are many views regarding which diet is ideal, so I decided to include some of the information from my book *Feasting and Fasting*. But please don't get caught up in the *diet craze*. The reason most diets don't work is because a short-term solution (dieting) cannot fix a long-term problem (obesity). Focus on how God designed you and eat accordingly. Stay active and consume foods in moderation. Make health a priority as well as a lifestyle.

Vegans, vegetarians, proponents of plant-based diets, and meat promoters all argue that their diet is best. Throw the raw diet crowd into the mix, and the confusion only increases. Many of these diets overlap but with some stark differences. For example, hard-core raw advocates don't cook any food. They consume it straight from the tree, vine, or ground. Plant-based diets promote raw, but they are often flexible and have a much broader range of choices.

I don't claim to have all the answers; even experts in the field of nutrition are divided, but we can glean a great deal from the biblical account. So let's begin where God begins.

> "In the beginning of creation, God said: 'Behold, I have given you every plant yielding seed that is on the surface of all the earth, and every tree which has fruit yielding seed; it shall be food for you; and to every beast of the earth and to every bird of the sky and to every thing that moves on the earth which has life, *I have given every green plant for food*'; and it was so" (Gen. 1:29–30 NASB; *italics* mine).

It's clear that we were designed to eat living, plant-based food. The life of the plant via vitamins, minerals, phytochemicals, fiber, and enzymes are to be deposited into the body—to restore, renew, and replenish. Ironically, when we eat whole plant-based foods, we often don't have to be as watchful regarding calories.

THE PLANT PROTEIN DEBATE

I'm not a fan of the idea that we need to consume a ton of protein. Yes, keto and paleo diets have their place, but I don't believe that some forms of those diets are the healthiest options, especially long-term. Care must be taken on these diets to eat an abundance of veggies and fiber.[2] Sure, you may find stories of Eskimos living on fish in the barren north (and most people do consume too many carbohydrates), but if we look at God's design, we see that plant-power is the way to go (there are plant-based keto diets).[3]

Sadly, many of those who promote these types of diets form their opinions based on the theory of *evolution*. But we must look at how we were *created* by a Creator, and start there.

With that said, I agree that many people don't consume enough of the *right* protein. For example, organic black beans have approximately seven to eight grams per half cup, and the fiber content is off the chart at around sixteen grams per cup. Talk about a superfood. I encourage you to do your own research on how plant food can sufficiently provide enough protein. More in the footnote.[4]

MANY QUESTIONS BUT FEW ANSWERS

After the great flood, meat consumption was introduced. Everything that lives and moves was to be food except the blood that is in the animal (Gen. 9:3). The blood of an animal contains toxins. Many diseases travel in the blood. God also identified clean and unclean animals. Unclean animals, such as pork, are still not considered healthy since viruses, bacteria, and parasites are easily transferred from the pig to us.

Was man not to consume meat until after the flood, approximately 1,600 years after the fall of man? If so, why? Did early man eat only plants for over 16 centuries before God allowed meat?[5] How did a plant-based diet provide enough calcium, iron, and zinc when they are difficult to obtain in a plant-based diet? Is it permissible to eat meat and dairy but not ideal? Should it be consumed sparingly? Does it balance nature (kill and eat)?

As you can see, we have a lot of questions and not too many solid answers.

MY PERSONAL VIEW ON THE BEST DIET

Biblically speaking, you can find support for a few different views, but I know from my own experience that I feel much better when meat and dairy consumption, along with processed food, is minimal. Although I blow it from time to time, I focus on eating lower calorie, nutrient-dense foods. Ironically, they are finding that this type of calorie restriction can lead to longevity. I'm not advocating a calorie counting diet; I'm simply suggesting that we consume whole, nutrient-dense plant foods when we *need* to instead of eating when we *want* to. Limit snacking throughout the day as well.[6] The old adage is true: *Eat half, walk double, laugh triple, and love without measure.*

I know it's not what many of us want to hear (I love meat), but consuming dead, decaying flesh over a long period of time, as well sugar and junk food, can wreak havoc on the body—from colon cancer to heart disease and from chronic inflammation to obesity—meat and dairy contain certain compounds that feed disease, even if they are organic.[7] Increased levels of sugar intake, along with a substantial rise in meat or dairy consumption, could be one possible link to cancer. It's the one-two punch. Dr. Joel Fuhrman has noted this as well (see footnote).[8]

In short, high sugar intake releases insulin into the bloodstream, and high levels of animal protein consumption can raise *insulin-like growth factor 1* (IGF-1). IGF-1 is a hormone that is similar to insulin. It joins with *growth hormone* to reproduce and regenerate cells. *This is great news if the cells are healthy but bad news if they are cancerous.* Excess sugar sparks the flame of disease, and the abundant IGF-1 throws gas on the fire.

On the other hand, as I just said, life-giving plant-food places vitamins, minerals, and powerful phytochemicals directly into the body that aid in recovery and immunity. There are many studies that show how a plant-based diet can reverse everything from heart disease to chronic inflammation, especially in conjunction with fasting.[9]

CONSIDER QUALITY AND QUANTITY

If you choose to eat meat and dairy, consider both the *quantity* and the *quality*. For example, if I eat meat or dairy, it's usually minimal and not very often (I like raw goat's milk on occasions). If the majority of our diet consists of whole, plant-based food with little meat and dairy, it won't affect health negatively in the same way that eating the standard American diet will.

The key is *moderation*, which means drinking or eating something *occasionally*. Unfortunately, moderation is often abused, and very unhealthy patterns develop. The apostle Paul said all things may be allowed, but all things are not beneficial (1 Cor. 10:23). In most areas where people live the longest, their diets are primarily plant-based.

I also believe that the pre-flood atmosphere of the earth was much different than our living conditions. Man lived in a healthier environment that may have provided more oxygen and greater protection against the harmful rays of the sun, and plants and fruit-bearing trees grew in abundance.

After the flood, however, fruits and vegetables became scarce (see Gen. 8:22; seedtime and harvest). I believe that God allowed meat consumption because of this scarcity. And keep in mind that meat and dairy were much cleaner than they are now, and people were much more active. Those two key factors are very significant. Not to mention the high fiber content of plant food;

fiber we desperately need to fight disease by helping to cleanse the colon.[10]

Personally, I'd rather err on the side of eating what we were designed to eat. The last chapter in the book of Revelation even talks about the *tree of life* providing fruit for the healing of the nations (Rev. 22:2). Interesting nonetheless.

Healthy meat and dairy can be enjoyed in moderation from time to time for those who want to go this route. But keep in mind that there's a big difference between organic grass-fed meat and processed luncheon meat preserved with sodium nitrates.

A FEW SCRIPTURES TO CONSIDER ABOUT FOOD

- In Ezekiel 4:9, we read that Ezekiel was to take "wheat, barley, beans, lentils, millet, and spelt" and make bread. This plant combination has many health benefits.
- In Deuteronomy 8:7-8, God said that He would bring them into a good land full of wheat and barley as well as figs, pomegranates, olive oil, and honey. And in Deuteronomy 20:19 God said that "the tree of the field is man's food."
- In Daniel 1, Daniel consumed vegetables and water for ten days and had great success in appearance and health.
- In Daniel 10, it appears that he did this again for twenty-one days. The spiritual outcome was incredible. I find it interesting that God blesses fasts where only vegetables are consumed. Meat aligns more with our animalistic nature. People were often rebuked because of gluttony, especially over meat (see Num. 11).
- When God fed the children of Israel in the wilderness,

He provided "bread from heaven" known as manna (Ex. 16:4; John 6:31). It had the appearance of bdellium (from trees). The Bible states the manna tasted like wafers made with honey. The perfect food that God chose appears to be plant-based, not meat-based. This is rather compelling for me. Then God brought in millions of quail because the people "lusted for meat."

- In Acts 10, we find that Peter had a vision in which God instructed him to kill and eat meat, but in context, God was using it as an example to minister to those who were not Jews.
- In Romans 14:1–2, the Apostle Paul talks about not judging a person who eats meat. But again, this could be referring to the unclean nature of certain foods and whether those foods were offered to idols rather than being a proof text for meat-based diets.

In 1 Timothy 4:3–4, Paul said that in the last days deceiving spirits will command people to abstain from certain foods—foods which God created to be received with thanksgiving. This verse is one reason why I don't prohibit any food that God created for food, including healthy meat and dairy. But it's also crystal clear that most people are not eating God-given food.

No wonder we experience so many emotional, physical, and mental problems that often affect our spiritual health.

KEY REMINDERS ABOUT FOOD

⇨ 1st REMINDER: Be careful when making absolute and dogmatic statements about food choices, but *healthy, clean plant-based foods* should be a high percentage of your diet. But if you struggle with being overweight, even "healthy" foods such as nuts and healthy oils should be consumed in moderation because of their high caloric content.

By clean, I mean eating organic when possible. *The Shoppers Guide to Pesticides in Produce* reveals a startling fact: "The average American eats about eight pounds of fresh strawberries a year—and with them, dozens of pesticides, including chemicals that have been linked to cancer and reproductive damage, or that are banned in Europe." It continues, "Non-organic strawberries tested by scientists at the Department of Agriculture in 2015 and 2016 contained an average of 7.8 different pesticides per sample, compared to 2.2 pesticides per sample for all other produce, according to EWG's analysis."[11]

Yes, eating organic produce can be more expensive, but isn't disease more costly? It will eventually bankrupt our nation. Save money by simply discontinuing many of your snacking stops at convenience stores and you can afford organic food. That simple change will easily save the average family hundreds of dollars a month. Also, consider buying certain things, like organic beans and nuts, in bulk. They are not more expensive in bulk when compared to non-organic. Items such as bananas and avocados don't need to be organic if you're on a tight budget.

Although I didn't touch on genetically modified food, be careful there too.

⇨ 2nd REMINDER: There has been a big movement away from focusing on the calorie content of healthy food, and I agree with most of the conclusions, but consuming more calories than you burn throughout the day will lead to weight gain. Granted, fluctuating hormone levels, along with the cell's ability to adapt to calorie restriction, complicates the process. Although it's wise to be aware of how many calories you're consuming, at least initially, there is no one-size-fits-all approach. I've talked to people who ate a lot of nuts and drank healthy juice, yet wondered why they weren't losing weight. In their case, they were consuming too many calories.

⇨ 3rd REMINDER: It's also wise to avoid adding salt to food while keeping an eye on oil usage. Consuming added sodium often makes us hungrier, and the extra calories in oil don't help our cause if one is trying to lose weight. I'm not suggesting to never use oil, but to be careful in the amount and the type of oil that is used. Refined oils, for example, are not healthy.

⇨ 4th REMINDER: Don't forget how important hydration is to overall health and digestion. It's not an accident that fruits and vegetables contain a great deal of water, some upwards of 90%. Dead food often has zero water content. I suggest drinking a *minimum* of a half-gallon of water a day.

If we add up everything that we have discussed so far, it's clear to see why *poor* food choices are causing *poor* health.[12] As Hippocrates once said, "Let food be thy medicine and medicine be thy food."

* See my book *Feasting and Fasting* for more on this topic.

DON'T MAKE THE SAME MISTAKE

We must be careful not to make the same mistake about *good* carbohydrates that we did about *healthy* fat in the 1980s and 1990s. Granted, there are some individuals who need to pay close attention to the amount of healthy carbohydrates they consume, but the right type of carbohydrates, like the right type of fats, are good and God-given in moderation for most of us.

The healthiest people on the planet eat primarily plant-based carbohydrates, sometimes making it upwards of 80% of their diet.

They also have very different microbiomes as a result of a plant-based diet that seems to help with overall health.[13]

They are also more active and they often deal with stress better than we do here in the USA. Their food is clean and whole, and they are rarely overweight.

Sadly, it's been estimated that for the first time in two centuries, the current generation of children in America may have shorter life expectancies than their parents. And they've been saying this for over a decade.[14] Little has changed.

If we eat God's food, move more, deal with stress His way, get enough sleep, and seek God daily, poor food choices now and then shouldn't affect us nearly as severely as they do when not following this checklist.

Choose wisely, and don't make the same mistake as countless Americans, because once you make a choice, it then makes you.

A MUST-READ FASTING EXPERIENCE

With so much going on in our nation, I knew that my fast needed to be monumental. There was, and still is, too much at stake.

With mass shootings, debilitating civil unrest and the rapid collapse of God-given freedoms, along with the *cancel culture's* attack on Christians and the passing of ungodly legislation, as well as a multitude of other concerns, I knew that my fast needed to be monumental and powerful. There was, and still is, too much at stake.

Although I hope that my experience will help you personalize your own fasting experience, I don't recommend following what I did. In general, the faster's physical condition, experience, supervision, and health all play a role in determining the length of a fast. Don't fret—God will meet you right where you are. Take time and pray for wisdom, direction, and confirmation. Begin by missing a meal or two, then try a whole day and build on that. Instead of eating at those times, open the Word, pray, and seek the heart of God.

In my case, God had been dealing with me for a few years regarding a lengthy fast, but I kept saying, "No way! That's impossible. I lead a church, manage our radio network, write articles for Christian publications, and I'm married with five kids." But after our elder board granted me a sabbatical at the end of January 2021, I thought, "Here is my chance to finally fast longer than normal"—not knowing that this *fasting sabbatical* would be one of the hardest things that I've ever done. I failed a few times along the way and almost gave up. Those seasons of failure were very humbling.

Additionally, although my purpose was for spiritual reasons, I also felt that God wanted me to lose weight. Although most wouldn't think that I needed to lose weight at 6' 2" and 222 pounds, the fact is that I did. An ideal weight for my height is anywhere between 170 and 190. Viewing footage from the 1950s to the 1970s shows that most Americans were slender. What happened?

As men, we've been slowly conditioned over the years to think that bigger means better. Trust me, that's not the case. Being one of the biggest and strongest guys in my area around the year 1990, made this a hard pill for me to swallow for many years. Every now and then, I see a picture of me over 270 pounds on the internet and I cringe. I was strong on the outside, but my heavy weight, along with alcohol and steroids were damaging my body from the inside. It's been estimated that for every pound of fat we gain, our body makes up to seven new miles of blood vessels. Yes, you heard me correctly. Extra weight is hard on the human body.[1]

Over the last few years, I was also struggling with inflammation in my right knee and elbow, as well as in both shoulders. My lower back also bothered me most of my adult life, my eyesight was fading when I read small fonts, and my blood pressure was slowly increasing each year. All of these things improved tremendously while fasting.

I'm also at greater risk of developing health-related illnesses as I age; therefore, it was clear that it was time for a lengthy fast for both physical and spiritual reasons. An old proverb reads, "The illness that cannot be cured by fasting, cannot be cured by anything else." Regretfully, many don't know how true that statement is.

THE PHYSICAL CHALLENGES

I knew that it was going to be a difficult battle, but I wasn't prepared for all that transpired. I had to keep my eyes focused on my prayers for my kids, wife, church, and country, as well as the desire to experience breakthroughs in other areas. Too much was on the line, especially when I knew that God had called me to this season of fasting. Granted, the *length* of a fast isn't as important as the *heart* behind the fast, and sometimes we don't know how long to fast, but it often takes time for spiritual breakthroughs to occur as we wrestle against opposition (cf. Ephesians 6, Daniel 10:13, and Mark 9:29).

Looking back, I probably could have maintained my work schedule most of the time. In one sense, even though busyness wasn't the goal of the fast and should be avoided, it would have been easier to fast while working. Spending a great deal of time at home had its challenges—from warm sourdough bread dripping with grass-fed butter to homemade treats and temptation—food was everywhere. The aroma of cooked organic grass-fed meat and garlic bread wafted through our home on a few occasions.

Not only was boredom, temptation, and my stomach against me, but so was my Type A go, go, go personality. Fasting is all about *slow, slow, slow,* not *go, go, go*. Fasting also increases spiritual warfare; so I had to deal with that as well. The enemy didn't want me to complete the fast or write this book.

Additionally, most people aren't fans of fasting, so I had to avoid the critics and the naysayers. Initially, I also had to avoid gatherings that involved food. Fellowship is an incredible gift, but difficult when one is called to a protracted season of fasting, prayer, reflection, and solitude.

It was difficult being distant from friends and family for a season, but there are times when you have to give up the *good* to focus on the *best*. I was excited about the completion so I could share with them why I was distant and isolated during this crucial time.

The times of refeeding were also very challenging. In many ways, they were harder than the fasts. With fasting, your mind is set and your resolve is steadfast, but with re-feeding, hunger is always whispering: "When can we eat again? What about now? How long do we have to wait? One more meal won't hurt." It takes great restraint to keep hunger at bay after ending a fast.

THE ROUGH ROAD AHEAD

I began my first attempt at a lengthy fast on January 17th; a week before my sabbatical began. By God's grace, even with a busy schedule, I made it through that week until I took a trip. I thought that I could maintain my fast while on the road, but the stress of snowy conditions proved me wrong. Once I returned home, I had to start all over again. I was discouraged and disappointed until I made up my mind to practice what I preach and *fall forward*.

I had a few more ups and downs and fasted here and there before I resolved to fast again, only to fail three days into it. As you can see, *the struggle is real*. Clearly, this was going to be a battle! Thoughts of doubt, fear, and failure were deeply embedded in my mind. I was also tired of feeling lousy, and not being able to do much because of how I felt while fasting.

Thankfully, there were positives in the midst of my failures. My wife and I were able to spend hours of quality time together, and I took two of my kids snowboarding. A nagging cough that I had for many weeks disappeared after two days of fasting drinking only water. I also noticed that I was more patient and understanding (cf. Galatians 5). I was able to spend more time reading God's Word and other books such as *Disciplines of a Godly Man*, *The Biography of John Bunyan*, and *The Science and Art of Fasting*. All of this provided momentum for the following fasting experience.

TAKING THE PLUNGE

With failure and frustration behind me, I finally took the plunge and began a prolonged water-only fast on the evening of March 16th, 2021. After missing approximately 100 plus meals and tons of snacks, treats, and temptations, it concluded on April 17th. Granted, I didn't do things perfectly, and I had to make a few adjustments (keep reading to find out more).

Although there were significant ups and downs during the journey, most of the time, I had never felt better both spiritually and physically. Although fasting has its own set of discomforts, it's amazing how much better you feel when you're not bloated or tired. With God's help, controlling my cravings rather than allowing my cravings to control me was very freeing.

My weight was approximately 222 pounds before the fast and dropped to 192 pounds after the fast. Again, although weight loss isn't the primary goal in a spiritual fast, it can be a blessing. God wants us to take care of our body, and when we benefit spiritually we also often benefit physically.

There were many times, however, when I had to move forward both physically and spiritually despite how I felt. From bad moods to low energy levels, it was a rollercoaster ride at times. For a few days, I would be doing great, but then a desire to quit and eat would overcome me. I wasn't necessarily hungry, I just wanted the fast to be over. But the following morning, I would be back on cloud nine. Talk about a rollercoaster ride.

To get me through the ups and downs, I gauged success by *commitment* rather than by *feelings*. I also focused on some of the spiritual and physical benefits:

Stronger faith
Deeper intimacy with God
Answered prayers
More energy
Ideal weight
Improved mobility
More patient and kind
Cleansing of body and soul

God truly strengthened me according to Isaiah 40:29, "He gives power to the weak, and to those who have no might He increases strength." But I also had a responsibility to say *no* and make the *right* choice. We can't always avoid temptation, but we can endure it with God's help. He will not allow us to be tempted beyond what we can handle (cf. 1 Corinthians 10:13).

DID I EAT OR DRINK ANYTHING?

Throughout the fast, I drank water . . . lots of water; however, as stated earlier, I didn't fast perfectly. There were times when I took in nutrients as noted below:

1) *Speaking Engagement*: Approximately two weeks into the fast, I traveled to a church in Southern California to film an interview on Saturday and give a brief exhortation at all three Sunday services (see the footnote).[2] Talk about a full weekend. When I felt weak, I couldn't go back to the hotel twenty minutes away and rest. I had to fulfill my responsibilities and commitments. So I decided to eat to get through that day, but I had to deny many things that weekend.

For instance, it was very challenging having water for lunch at a nice restaurant with pastor Rob McCoy and his wife. And I ordered nothing when my wife had dinner at California's famous In-and-Out Burger, or when the hotel served an incredible Eggs Benedict breakfast along with an array of other temptations. As a result of denying all of these things, the weekend was a complete success. God honored and blessed it more than I could have imagined. Granted, if I knew for certain that God wanted me to press through regardless of how I felt, then I would have done so, but I had to use wisdom.

2) *Time with my Daughter*: Another time when I ate was when I took my daughter on a long bike ride on her birthday. We easily burned 1,000 calories after riding nearly an hour and a half. Recall what I previously stated about gluconeogenesis: If I didn't consume anything for the ride I would have used a great deal of muscle for fuel and possibly done more harm than good as well as hinder healing. Plus, I wouldn't have been able to go on the bike ride due to low energy levels.

My daughter had been looking forward to this day for over a month. Temporarily altering my fast meant the world to her. I was back to consuming water only in the morning. We all have different circumstances, situations, and goals. Spending the day with my daughter outweighed staying at home. *Your reset needs to be both practical and doable.* Although it would be ideal, most of us can't totally disengage for forty days when we have kids and responsibilities.

Throughout the *fasting sabbatical*, I had to say no to everything from incredible homemade dinners to superb Mexican food lunches, and from my favorite healthy chocolate muffins to homemade peanut butter cookies. I also drank water each time we celebrated birthdays. At one of the party's, *Krispy Kreme* donuts called my name for over five hours. It wasn't fun.

I will also never forget when my daughter cooked organic lemon chicken pasta with alfredo sauce for dinner on Easter. The smell hit me like a freight train when I walked in the front door. I had to take a drive while they ate (the sense of smell is heightened when fasting).

The *fasting sabbatical* was a time of denial unlike anything I've ever experienced before, but boy was it worth it. As stated earlier: Perseverance is strengthened in the furnace of affliction and in the midst of defeat. Staying the course in spite of difficulties, obstacles, and discouragement (or when we cave in) is challenging, but well worth it. We come out of the battle stronger.

PAYING THE PRICE

Some of the comments I heard along the way, especially during phase two, were, "You're too skinny!," and, "Is everything okay—are you sick?" Or, "Why get so extreme? Is it really worth it?" If you're thinking the same thing, I will answer with what I said earlier: *There is simply too much at stake.* As a nation, it's clear that we are dying spiritually. Mass shootings are increasing, the suicide rate is escalating, and hopelessness is prevailing. I'd say that all of that is pretty extreme. So, you tell me, is it worth it?

Look at what we are leaving our children. I'm not sure what to say if that doesn't motivate all of us to pray and fast. Nothing has changed. Extreme problems demand extreme measures. The church has always fasted and prayed for God's favor, wisdom, and direction, as well as to prepare our hearts. In the same way that we cannot produce a bumper crop by making it rain, a spiritual awakening cannot be planned, but you can till the soil of your heart. God said that He will "revive the spirit of the lowly" as well as "the heart of the contrite" (Isaiah 57:15).

The truth is that many are not willing to humble themselves and pay the price. When spiritual awakenings spread across our landscape, Christians spent countless hours praying and fasting. They paid the price. Will you?

FINAL FASTING RESULTS

Over a three-month period, I water fasted for forty days. Although the physical aspects of a fast are not the priority, they are important. My blood pressure dropped from 130/90 to 115/75. My average pulse rate dropped from approximately 75 beats a minute to 60, then the 50s. Apparently, my heart received a good rest.

Throughout this time, all my kids came down with colds, but I never came down with anything like I normally would. Fasting allows the body to attack infections at a greater intensity because all of the energy is focused on overcoming the intruder rather than digesting and processing food.

I felt like the fast cleansed my entire body—all my organs profited. The experience was life-changing, both physically and spiritually. I wrote this book, renewed my relationship with the Lord, improved my relationship with my wife and kids, and many prayers were answered in profound ways. I also came back from my sabbatical fully refreshed. I call that a successful fast.

Although I didn't completely refrain from looking at the media, I scaled back considerably and didn't read 99% of the comments, threads, or responses on social media. It was very refreshing. You should try it.

Even though there were challenging days, the spiritual benefits were amazing as well.

Special Note: If you're curious how I'm doing after the fast and if the results were maintained, make sure to subscribe to my YouTube channel. Depending on when you're reading this, I'm hoping to give an update in the summer of 2021, but there are plenty of videos in the archives covering a variety of topics.

THE POWER OF THE MADE-UP MIND

If you don't control what you think you'll never control what you do. An unhealthy mindset is like a flat tire. You're not going anywhere until you change it.

The mind controls just about everything we do, so it's no surprise that success is mainly found in the power of the made-up mind and renewed thinking. This is why the next section, *Daily Reflections,* focuses on renewing the mind through reading and applying biblical principles. Romans 12:2 spells it out clearly: "And do not be conformed to this world, but be transformed by the renewing of your mind, that you may prove what is that good and acceptable and perfect will of God."

The lethargic spiritual condition of many today simply reflects our lack of passion for God. While potlucks and fellowship around food have their place, they aren't going to cut it in these dire times. We also need extended times of prayer, fasting, and worship to renew the mind. Unplug the TV and the PC and begin seeking God like never before.

HUNGER FOR GOD IS THE MOTIVATION

If you would receive $10,000 following a week-long fast drinking just water would you do it? No doubt the motivation to earn the money would outweigh the difficulties of the fast. Shouldn't our hunger for God motivate us more than money? Success begins in the mind. *If you don't control what you think you'll never control what you do.* An unhealthy mindset is like a flat tire. You're not going anywhere until you change it.

Decide early what you'd like to do over the next forty days, and stay the course. Some readers may fast here and there, while others may change their diet altogether and fast intermittently, while others may attempt a lengthy fast. Determine in your mind to seek God as you step out in faith.

Are you ready to reset your life and begin your forty-day journey? If you made it this far, I believe that you are, but remember, it's not about perfection, but direction. Keep moving forward despite setbacks. Don't let discouragement and failure stand in your way. Get back up and keep fighting. God's not done with you yet. Find strength in Him. Make up your mind today to see it through. We must first discipline ourselves then results will follow.

As I've said many times before: I could write an entire book on my failures, but instead, I try to follow the Apostle Paul's advice, and I encourage you to do the same: *"Forgetting those things which are behind and reaching forward to those things which are ahead"* (Philippians 3:13). Forget your past mistakes, but remember the lessons learned because of them. We overcome the pain of regret by allowing God to rebuild our life. Though the road ahead may be uncertain at times, the solid ground beneath will never shift. It's all about Who you know.

PART TWO

DAILY REFLECTIONS

DAY ONE

HOW TO REST IN TURBULENT TIMES

From the COVID crisis to financial burdens, and from fear and isolation to a divided nation, millions are lacking peace and rest. But I believe we can find rest if we look to the right source. Expending energy has a time and a very important place in our lives—we were created to work, but we were also created to rest. The problem for many is that they never stop, rest, renew, and refocus. They are always wound up, so to speak.

Whether it's running the kids back and forth seven days a week or working frantic hours, we are busier than ever because we often measure success by busyness. *The busier I am, the more successful I am*, so we think.

In a helpful article on the reasons spiritual leaders need rest (which all of us should read), author Cary Schmidt says, "Pastors and ministry leaders don't ever really 'clock out.' It's a part of the call. The needs are incessant. The only means of real survival is to pull away from the demands long enough to restore. Everyone must come up for air eventually or die."[1] Nowadays, most of us never "clock out."

Schmidt adds, "The primary reason we struggle to rest is that our identity is tied to the things that keep us running at a breakneck pace. We have anchored our sense of self to what we do *for God*—therefore we can never do enough, and if we stop (even for a short time), we feel a loss of self and fear His disapproval."

Although his comments are mainly directed to pastors, could it be that God wants many of us to slow down? Absolutely. We are glued to screens, addicted to phones, and enslaved to sports and entertainment. We scurry around looking for the next thing to do. We go to bed exhausted and wake up exhausted. Something must change. Are you ready to get started? If so, what things can you remove today and this week that are draining your spiritual tanks? As just a few examples, I found it very helpful to turn *off* the social media notifications on my phone. That way I control them versus them controlling me. I also put the phone away (when I can) instead of always having it by me. I also don't look at it an hour before going to bed. These three simple changes helped a great deal.

⇒ How about you? What simple changes can you begin making today? A long journey begins with the first step.

DAY TWO

ARE YOU SPIRITUALLY HEALTHY?

There are many signs of spiritual health such as the proclamation of truth, community outreach, spiritual growth, and so on, but powerful prayer should top the list. This will be my focus.

Every year, I try to spend a few days alone in a cabin to slow down, reflect, and pray—to renew my mind. The importance of time alone with God is invaluable. Renewal begins and ends with prayer. Spiritually speaking, it has been said that when we cease to pray, we cease to live.

To renew means "to reestablish something after an interruption." Life can easily interrupt fellowship with God. We are renewed through prayer and time alone with Him. As a matter of biblical fact, mighty fillings of the Spirit often occurred after extended times of prayer and repentance.

During these times of retreat, I'm often reminded that the overall spiritual condition of my heart will be a reflection of my prayer life. E.M. Bounds believed that without prayer in the pulpit, "The church becomes a graveyard, not an embattled army. Praise and prayer are stifled; worship is dead. The preacher and the preaching encourages sin, not holiness . . . preaching which kills is prayerless preaching. Without prayer, the preacher creates death, and not life."

You may ask, "What does this have to do with me? I'm not a pastor!" It has everything to do with you! Powerful, heartfelt prayer moves the hand of God.

William Bramwell, a powerful Methodist circuit rider, often spent hours a day on his knees to sustain his preaching. It was not uncommon for the great Scottish preacher, John Welch, who died in 1622, to spend hours in prayerful sermon preparation. Robert Murray M'Cheyne, one of Scotland's most anointed preachers, was a powerful man of prayer. The Puritans, as the result of much prayer, produced some of the greatest writings and devotional material that the church has ever known. And, I am sure, this can be said of anointed writers today. Prayer is the first sign of spiritual health.

⇒ How are you doing in this area? If prayer is lacking, put it on your calendar and begin today.

DAY THREE

HOW ARE YOU MEASURING SUCCESS?

Noted author and speaker, Josh McDowell, once said, "One of the most common questions I get is, 'How can we live for Christ, when we don't want the Christ that our parents have'?" What a powerful question.

A few decades ago, being a devoted parent was viewed as the most important job one could have. Qualities such as honesty, integrity, commitment, discipline, and a strong work ethic are not easily taught; they are instilled through lives that model these traits. Never underestimate the power of parenting—even if you are a single parent!

If you're not a parent and don't have any children, it's still important to ask, "How am I measuring success?" Make no mistake about it, we live in a society that emphasizes wealth and what we possess. We fail to remember that these things have no lasting value. I don't remember my father's income or many of the physical things my parents gave to me. I do, however, remember the values they taught . . . those things that money cannot buy. They taught that success is not measured by what we have, but rather by what we give. It's been well stated: "The best things in life aren't things."

It's possible to succeed in business, ministry, and other endeavors, but fail at home. Look around, it's happening everywhere, from the pulpit to the boardroom. Unfortunately, the price of success is often paid at the expense of the family.

A friend once relayed a tragic story. He told of a trip to the hospital to visit a man who was dying. The man could no longer speak; however, he could write. His desire was to be taken off life-support, but what followed was more devastating. The man cried as he wrote that he regretted that he had not spent more time with his family. He was in anguish over the fact that he had not been a better father, but instead, had built his life around other things.

When all is said and done, it is devastating to find that life was invested in those things that hold no lasting value. Don't give your children a self-help book or a lecture, or simply drop them off at church, but more importantly, regardless of their age, have your children desire the Christ they see in you. This is the true measure of success.

⇒ How are you doing in this area? What things need to be re-prioritized, and how will you go about doing it? Often, we have to remove or minimize distractions before we can elevate more important things.

DAY FOUR

WHY HAVE I LOST MY PASSION FOR LIFE?

As a pastor, I often hear, "I've lost my passion. What's going on?" Responses differ depending on the situation, but one thing is clear: Our passion and purpose, along with obedience to God, are closely interwoven. Problems arise when we seek comfort, convenience, money, status, or recognition above seeking God and what He desires for us. Purpose is found in doing God's will God's way.

Literally millions of men are unhappy simply because they chose a lucrative career rather than a career that they were gifted for and enjoy. They put God's will on the back burner and wonder why they lack passion. Likewise, countless women are unhappy because they allow the world's mindset to influence them. Being a stay-at-home mother was once prized and cherished; today, it's frowned upon.

If life is all about us and what we want, we will always struggle with discouragement. We need to recognize that there is a Master Builder who has a plan. How do you avoid the emotional roller coaster? First, check the obvious (I will be revisiting these often throughout the book): Who are you associating with? What do you watch and/or listen to? Does it build you up spiritually, or pull you down? What thoughts fill your mind? Are they negative, bitter thoughts, or thankful thoughts? Are you walking in obedience to God's Word? If not, "the way of transgressors is hard" (Prov. 13:15). Start here.

Mild depression and sadness are common to all of us, but when it lingers, it often requires more focused attention. Exercise, fun, friendship, forgiveness, kindness—all are biblical solutions that can lead to joy. There are clear cases of clinical depression that I'm not simply dismissing, but our first step must be complete abandonment to God. A fully surrendered life that focuses on His Word and His promises will never lead you in the wrong direction. Fulfilling our purpose in life is not a destination; it's a journey through day-to-day opportunities. It can be filled with unforeseen challenges, but it's a rewarding journey if you look to the Creator to provide the compass.

Secondly, are you a critical person? It's hard to be joyful when you're critical. First Thessalonians 5:16-19 says: "Rejoice always, pray without ceasing, give thanks in all circumstances; for this is the will of God in Christ Jesus for you. Do not quench the Spirit."

Thirdly, are you truly obeying God's Word? James 1:22 tells us that we live in deception if we only hear God's Word without applying it to our lives. Disobedience leads to deception, and deception often leads to depression.

Finally, are you allowing circumstances to affect your joy? Many are happy when life goes their way, but very unhappy when it does not. This is largely because they measure happiness by what's happening to them. When things go well, they're happy, when things go poorly, they're unhappy. I'm not suggesting that we should never be upset or depressed, but if happiness is measured by our circumstances, it's going to be a very rough road ahead.

⇒ Are you spending time in prayer asking for direction? What about spending time reading the Bible to discern God's will and to obey it? If you're critical, judgmental, and angry, take time now and repent. Also, memorize Romans 15:13 this week, "May the God of hope fill you with all joy and peace as you trust in him, so that you may overflow with hope by the power of the Holy Spirit."

DAY FIVE

WHAT GOES IN COMES OUT

One thing that amazes me is how far we have drifted in our entertainment choices—going from *Leave it to Beaver* and *I Love Lucy* a generation ago, to media choices that are dark, demonic, perverted, and hypersexual today, and we wonder why we are so depressed, fearful, and lost.

Ponder these three points in light of your current entertainment choices:

1. There is no such thing as good magic, good witches, or pleasant darkness. These things, by their very nature, are evil. Scripture makes it clear that fascination with the powers of darkness, sexuality, and the occult has no place in the heart or the mind of a Christian. Our minds are to be fixed on what is noble, pure, excellent, and good (Philippians 4:8). Jesus never encouraged enthusiasm over things that God forbade. There are no scriptural grounds in defense of these types of media choices. It's more reasonable for Christians who enjoy these movies to simply admit that they enjoy them, rather than try to defend them.

2. We must be pure vessels that God can use (2 Timothy 2:19-21.) A pure vessel cannot come from a polluted mind. Again, enchantments, witchcraft, familiar spirits, idolatry, and sexual perversion are always condemned as evil practices throughout the Bible. For example, 2 Chronicles 33:6 says that those who use enchantments and witchcraft, and who deal with familiar spirits and wizards, provoke the Lord to anger. There is no gray area here. If these things entertain, something is clearly wrong. Darkness should not entertain, and sexual perversion should not fascinate us. Once something entertains us, we then accept it. Once accepted, it begins to influence. *Sin fascinates before it assassinates.*

3. Being selective with what we watch and listen to has nothing to do with legalism; it has everything to do with wisdom. We are to recognize what glorifies Christ and what does not, and then choose accordingly. It's not about following rules. Let your freedom in Christ, and a relationship with Him, guide you. We've all watched questionable material and have made wrong choices; don't live with ongoing regret. But don't justify wrong behavior by thinking that God doesn't care about what you watch or listen to, because He does; we serve and love God with our mind (cf. Romans 7:25).

This message is not a small recommendation, it's a call to a life-changing decision. What goes in the mind ultimately comes out in our actions. Why walk willingly into the enemy's camp? Why quench and grieve the Spirit of God? It's impossible to develop a deep respect and desire for God if we repeatedly fill our minds with things that oppose Him.

⇒ Let me leave you with this thought: Are you willing to do what it takes to protect your mind and your relationship with the

Lord? It's your choice. Drawing a line can be out of step with the mainstream, but, like Joshua, we too must say, "Choose this day whom you will serve as for me and my house, we will serve the Lord" (Joshua 24:15).

DAY SIX

TRUTH–A HILL ON WHICH TO DIE

A weapon of destruction has set its sights on our nation, our homes, and our families. Cultural constructs such as relativism and postmodernism defiantly challenge the truth, but they will ultimately lead to destruction. Attacking absolute truth is like a ship waging war on a lighthouse; it can't win. It will destroy the very thing that is designed to guide it to safety. Truth cannot be negotiated, bargained with, or debated.

In battle, there are key strongholds that must be taken, or kept at all costs in order to win. These are "hills on which to die." Today, absolute truth is one such hill. To truly reset your life and experience God, truth must be foundational.

When people depart from absolute truth, and thus, quench and grieve the Spirit of God, they become mechanical in their approach to Christianity and lose the ability to truly hear from God. The word of God is not "in their hearts like a burning fire," but relative, powerless, and debatable. This is what we see today; many are not truly worshipping God, as Jesus said, "in spirit and in truth." Christians are to be pillars who support truth, not those who oppose it.

Unfortunately, those who are sounding the alarm are often categorized as irrational, judgmental, bigoted, and intolerant. But how can we warn if we won't confront? We are not called to make truth tolerable, but to make it clear.

How are you doing in this area of truth? Are you fully embracing God's absolute truth? If not, take time today and make that commitment, or recommitment, to the truth. It's the only sure foundation on which we should build our lives. The key is to spend significant time in God's Word. This simple change will transform your mind by renewing it with the truth. *Times may change but truth does not change.*

⇒ In order to apply the truth, you must first know what the truth is. Commit to reading thirty minutes of God's Word each day from a good study Bible.[1] Then, throughout the day, apply what you have learned. In the morning and evening, instead of looking at the news and social media, read and pray. Turn off all electronics an hour before bed and read a good book instead. Close with prayer and reflection.

DAY SEVEN

THE DESPERATE NEED FOR GENUINE WORSHIP

Most who attend church are not truly worshipping God—they are simply going through the motions. Those who have truly experienced God worship Him. Worship is a byproduct of genuine faith. Worship, in the truest sense of the word, is a lifestyle of worship and not just participating in corporate singing. Our lifestyle should reflect a heart of worship. This is not optional, it's vital.

We cannot live like hell all week and expect heaven to come. We cannot fill our minds with darkness all week and expect the light of Christ to shine during worship. We cannot worship ourselves, and things, all week and expect to turn our affections toward God on one designated day. What we watch and listen to affects the heart—it's impossible to separate the two. For example, if a Christian fills their mind with the world all week and expects to worship God on Sunday, they will be gravely mistaken. "The gratification of the flesh and the fullness of the Spirit do not go hand in hand" (R.A. Torrey). What goes in ultimately comes out.

Genuine worship must begin with a desire for holiness, and a desire to be in the presence of God. Worship is warfare: "You have to wrestle against the things that prevent you from getting to God" (Oswald Chambers).

For those who say, "I'm too busy to cultivate a life focused on worship," you may want to re-think that. Contrary to what many think, a devotional life centered around worship actually helps with the utilization of time. Worshipful devotion aids in discipline, patience, peace, and joy.

What distracts you? What zaps your time, energy, and resources? Time, like money, is multiplied when we give first to God. Social life, business life, and personal life all benefit from making worship a priority. If we are too busy to worship God—we are too busy!

Genuine worship also generates heartfelt forgiveness and reconciliation. In Matthew 5:24, Jesus encourages us to fix broken relationships before worshipping. Why is this a key ingredient to genuine worship? In short, critical, divisive people who do not forgive or release bitterness, anger, and hurt, never experience freedom, happiness, or true worship. Worship is often hindered as the result of past pain and resentment. The act of true worship from a grateful heart is impossible when these conditions exist. Pain can prevent worship or propel you to it. The choice is yours.

Ephesians 4:31-32 reminds us, "Let all bitterness, wrath, anger, clamor, and evil speaking be put away from you, with all malice. And be kind to one another, tenderhearted, forgiving one another, even as God in Christ forgave you." Simply stated, bitterness, negativity, and anger hinder genuine worship. Take the time now and repent of these destructive attitudes if they exist. Call or write those who have offended you; asking for forgiveness (if warranted) or restoration, especially spouses (or ex-spouses).

Ask God to help you remove those things that hinder your relationship with Him. It is in the living and giving of genuine worship that we are transformed. Don't run from it, run to it!

⇒ Start by replacing secular music with Christian music that you enjoy and that is doctrinally sound. Begin and end your day with listening and praying. But again, worship isn't just about singing; it involves every aspect of our lives. Make it your goal to know Christ more deeply.

DAY EIGHT

WORSHIP—THE THERMOMETER OF THE HEART

Springboarding off of the previous reflection, the Hebrew for worship means to "bow down," or to "prostrate oneself." Worship is a posture reflecting homage and reverence toward the one true and living God. If there is a problem with worshipping God, the problem isn't with God, the problem is with us.

Worship serves as the thermometer of the heart by measuring our spiritual condition. Are we hot, cold, or lukewarm? Granted, worship isn't necessarily measured by actions such as jumping up and down; it's measured by the condition (temperature) of our heart—is it rejoicing for joy and submitting to God?

Sadly, many confuse false worship with genuine worship. According to numerous theological resources, false worship is when an entity, person, or object is worshipped instead of God— our passion for "something" outweighs our passion for Him; it draws us away. Most don't have idols on the shelf because they are parked in the garage. We don't pay homage to a statue in the living room because we are memorized by a 44" box affectionately known as "the entertainment center." We don't sacrifice things on the altar, but we do sacrifice our time (and time with our children) on the altar of misguided priorities.

Of course cars, televisions, and the Internet are not evil, they are neutral, but it is our love for them that tilts the scale away from God. We find hours a day for entertainment but have little time to worship. Do we honestly believe that this misapplication of priorities doesn't affect our spirituality? Think again.

False worship also includes inappropriate and improper acts supposedly directed toward God. Many simply go through the motions at church. They attend as if they are doing God a favor. The heart is not engaged and the soul is not lifted up. They are bored. Here is a test to measure the spiritual condition of the heart: Do we want the worship time to hurry and finish? Are we dreading another song as our eyes glance at the clock? Do we come late to miss the *boring* worship? If so, I would seriously encourage heart examination.

I am not suggesting that if the worship seems dead it's our fault; not all of the worship taking place is heartfelt and Spirit-led. Dry formalism and dead ritualism can be found in many churches. Many sing *about* God but they have never truly *experienced* Him —they have head knowledge without heart knowledge.

⇒ Is your worship thermometer reading cold? Simply adjust the thermostat and increase the heat through prayer, fasting, obedience, and worship. The choice is yours.

DAY NINE

THE BEGINNING OF WISDOM AND KNOWLEDGE

J.C. Ryle (1816-1900) once said that true Christians must stand guard as soldiers on enemy ground. The problem is that many love the world and do not fear God. They believe in heaven but they don't truly long for it. They "say" that they fear God but they don't live like it. They indulge in temptation rather than fight it. They enjoy sin rather than confront it. And they compromise rather than conquer. The lukewarm church disdains the heat of conviction. Holiness, to them, is outdated and the fear of the Lord is old-fashioned.

The present condition of our nation leaves one to wonder if the lack of the fear of the Lord is contributing to her spiritually dead condition: "I know your works: you are neither cold nor hot. Would that you were either cold or hot! So, because you are lukewarm, and neither hot nor cold, I will spit you out of my mouth . . ." (Revelation 3:15-17).

A healthy respect for God (fear) is what we desperately need. The fear of the Lord is mentioned frequently throughout the

Bible as the beginning of knowledge, wisdom, and understanding (cf. Proverbs 1:7; 9:10). Many feel that we should avoid mentioning the fear of the Lord because it makes people feel uncomfortable. Just writing that sentence makes me feel uncomfortable. "The Lord takes pleasure in those who fear Him" (Psalm 147:11). Joshua encouraged the people to "fear the Lord and serve him with all faithfulness" (24:14).

It's clear from Genesis to Revelation that we are to "serve the Lord with fear and rejoice with trembling" (Psalm 2:11). Jesus said, "Do not fear those who kill the body but cannot kill the soul. But rather fear Him who is able to destroy both soul and body in hell" (Matthew 10:28). Jesus spoke more on the fear of hell than on the glory of heaven. He thought it to be timely and urgent. "That makes me both love Him and fear Him! I love Him because He is my Savior, and I fear Him because He is my Judge" (A.W. Tozer).

Fearing the Lord isn't the type of fear one would have toward an abusive father, but rather, it's the type of fear that involves respect and reverence for God. For example, we fear jumping off a 100-story building because we respect gravity. Fear, in this sense, is good and God-given; it protects. It is also often through reverent fear that we come to Christ and redemption.

Society, as a whole, may have forgotten the fear of the Lord, but it doesn't follow that we should. Take time today and reflect on the awesomeness of God who commands the Oceans of the world, and in whose hands the destiny of nations are determined. "It is he who made the earth by his power, who established the world by his wisdom, and by his understanding stretched out the heavens" (Jeremiah 10:12 ESV). No army can overcome Him, no politician can overrule Him, and no nation can stop Him. Embrace God's wisdom today.

. . .

⇒ Mediate this week on Psalm 147:11, "The Lord takes pleasure in those who fear Him," as well as Psalm 31:19, "How great is Your goodness, which You have stored up for those who fear You." What stands out? How can you begin fearing the Lord?

DAY TEN

WHY DOESN'T SUCCESS SATISFY?

In celebration of Michael Jordan's 50th birthday some years back, ESPN senior writer Wright Thompson spent some time with M.J. Thompson gives the sense that Jordan isn't happy. "I would give up everything now to go back and play the game of basketball," Jordan laments. When asked how he copes with the devastating fact that he will never be who he was, Jordan states, "You don't. You learn to live with it."

Thompson continues, "Jordan might have stopped playing basketball, but the rage is still there. The fire remains, which is why he searches for release . . . the man has left the court, but the addictions won't leave the man."

This writer made a correct observation. Society tends to program our looks and actions. Women, as well as young girls, refer to magazines and TV to see how they should dress and act; teenage boys consult TV and the media for role models, and many men measure their self worth by what they have accomplished in business and financially, not realizing that a relationship with God, family, and others is the treasure they should be seeking.

Secular values have eroded qualities such as integrity, discipline, and commitment from our lives, just as water and time have eroded the banks of the Colorado River and left a vast Grand Canyon. Erosion can occur so slowly that we are unaware until its work is done. It has the power to change the course of a mighty river and it can surely change the course of our lives.

Don't allow a declining culture to erode essential qualities in your life. You can make a difference by following and obeying God's Word. With life, we were given power. The power to obey God is one of the greatest attributes that we possess. There is little we can do about life's glitches except to control the way that we respond to them. The obstacles ahead are not greater than God's power to take us through.

Most of us understand that money can buy the best mattress, but it can't guarantee sleep. Why do millionaires, movie stars, and top entertainers often turn to drugs and alcohol for the answers if success satisfies? Many discover that money, fame, and recognition are not the answers. CEOs, presidents, and vice presidents frequently admit that they are happy when they reach production goals, but very unhappy when under budget, largely because they measure happiness by what's happening to them. When things go well, they're happy, when things go poorly, they're unhappy. I'm not suggesting that we shouldn't be productive, but if happiness is measured by our circumstances, it's going to be a very rough road.

One of the happiest times in my life, for example, was when I went from running multiple fitness locations to making much less money digging ditches, writing, and managing nothing but my daily life. During this transition, I quickly learned that the more I owned, the more it owned me. Goals, dreams, and aspirations are God's desire for our lives, but when these things are based on self-gratification, we encounter problems emotionally, physically, and spiritually. Success doesn't satisfy us because we were not designed to be idols.

⇒ Jesus asked this question two thousand years ago and we are still asking it today: *What shall it profit any of us if we gain the whole world yet lose our soul?* (cf. Mark 8:36). Is there anything in between you and your relationship with Christ? Are you willing to remove it today?

DAY ELEVEN

RESETTING YOUR SITE ON THE TARGET

"Suicide has surpassed car crashes as the leading cause of injury death for Americans. Even more disturbing, in the world's greatest military, more U.S. soldiers died last year by suicide than in combat." David Kupelian wrote those words nearly a decade ago in his article, *Americans 'Snapping' by the Millions*.[1]

Kupelian continues, "Fully one-third of the nation's employees suffer chronic debilitating stress, and more than half of all 'millennials' (18 to 33-year-olds) experience a level of stress that keeps them awake at night, including large numbers diagnosed with depression or anxiety disorder."

Sadly, not much has changed. These statistics reveal that we are a nation adrift. We have lost our moral compass and we have rejected God. This departure has left our nation in a moral, as well as an emotional crisis. And this is exactly why we've seen mass shootings skyrocket. We've become a society focused on prosperity instead of provision, we value wealth instead of wisdom, and we are drawn to charisma instead of character. Our foundation as a nation, and as individuals, has slowly deteriorated. We are reaping what was sown years ago.

Please don't misunderstand, I'm not discounting the deep emotional and psychological pain associated with depression and anxiety, but I do want to remind you that God makes provision for all of our needs. There may be a time and a place for medication, but it should be the last resort, not the first. The first step must be toward God . . . toward a genuine relationship (more on this later).

Although not in all cases, depression is often a by-product of a misaligned heart. We consume food every day to live, why then, do we think that we can avoid worshipping the one true and living God and not die spiritually?

Proverbs 4:25-27 reminds us to look straight ahead and fix our eyes on what lies before us. Mark out a straight path for your feet and stick to it to stay safe. Don't get sidetracked. When I was a teen, my father would often take my brother and me "trap shooting." As soon as clay targets were released from a small building built partially underground, we'd pull the guns to our shoulders and prepare to fire. There were only seconds to aim and fire as the clay targets darted through the air. If we took our eyes off the target, even for a second, we would miss the shot. The same holds true for our spiritual lives. If we neglect to continually focus on the right path, we can miss the ultimate target—God's most productive plan for our lives.

A consistent theme found throughout the Bible is, "'Return to Me and worship Me,' says the Lord, 'and I will return to you. I will heal and restore. I will bind up the broken and strengthen the sick'" (cf. Zechariah 1:6; Ezekiel 34:16). The Lord is our only hope . . . our only cure. Jesus said, "Peace I leave with you; my peace I give you. I do not give to you as the world gives. Do not let your hearts be troubled and do not be afraid" (John 14:27).

⇒ Although I cover this topic in more detail on day thirty-seven, it's important to stop and reset your site on the target: Do you have this peace? Do you know the Prince of Peace? If not, you can change that; it all starts with having a vibrant relationship with the one true and living God.

DAY TWELVE

THIS WORD WILL SET YOU FREE

Believe it or not, over the years many Christians have sought to remove the word "repent" from Christianity. They said that we need to rethink our narrow view of the gospel and our restricted view of Biblical hermeneutics. Their rescripting seems ridiculous, but it's true. In reality, it's no surprise that they took this position—for Christianity to appear palatable and less intrusive to our culture, many feel that we need to rethink, redefine, and rename difficult truths, especially repentance.

I often preach about the desperate need for repentance—it's one of the hallmarks of my ministry. As a result, I'm often labeled "hard-core," "extreme," "un-loving," and "narrow-minded." But nothing could be further from the truth. I simply want to see people transformed by the power of God through repentance. Richard Owen Roberts states it well, "The Lord has been so deeply grieved by the refusal of the church to faithfully proclaim the whole counsel of His word in the power of the Holy Spirit that He has largely withdrawn from the church and left her to her own devices."[1]

Whether the word for repentance is *"nocham"* in the Old Testament, or *"metanoeō"* in the New Testament, biblical repentance involves turning from sin and turning to God—it's a condition of the heart. Acts 3:19 unapologetically confirms this: "Repent therefore and be converted, that your sins may be blotted out, so that times of refreshing may come from the presence of the Lord." Jesus said that "unless you repent you will all likewise perish" (Luke 13:5).

The influential Baptist evangelist, John R. Rice (1895-1980), said, "There is no way you can please God, no way you can have sweet communion with Him to get your prayers answered if you are in rebellion against the known will of God." Failing to turn from sin and turn to Christ results in rebellion against God.

When Mark 6:12 tells us that Jesus' disciples "went out and preached that people should repent," Jesus wasn't suggesting that the disciples rethink their narrow-mindedness, redefine their view of sin, or reinterpret the meaning of repentance. He was saying that people need to turn from sin and turn to God.

To suggest that everyone from the Old Testament prophets to Christ and the apostles, to the early church fathers and the reformers, to present-day scholars and theologians, misunderstood the real meaning of repentance, is the height of arrogance and deception. I would respect progressives more if they'd just say that they don't like the concept of repentance rather than trying to reinterpret its already crystal clear meaning.

Repentance is a true gift from God that affects everything in our lives. If our priorities, our passions, our goals, our dreams, and our desires are not changing—are we changing? I only say this because so many today have religion and not a true relationship with Christ. They are simply going through the motions. They have never truly repented. It's been said that if your religion has not changed your life, change your religion. Repentance is the one word that will set you free.

⇒ Are you making excuses and blaming others? Genuine repentance means that we own our sin. We're not sorry because we got caught, we're sorry because we wronged God and others. If you haven't done so yet, begin repairing relationships that were damaged as the result of unrepentant sin, including your relationship with God.

DAY THIRTEEN

EXPERIENCING GOD THROUGH HIS SPIRIT

The Holy Spirit is not some weird, mystical force. He is part of the triune nature of God. The Bible says that the Spirit intercedes, leads, guides, teaches, and so on (cf. Romans 8:26; Acts 8:29; John 16:13). He enables and empowers us to hunger and thirst for righteousness, and to boldly live for Christ. God's Word becomes living and active in the life of the believer who is continually filled with the Holy Spirit. Charles Spurgeon adds, "What can a hammer do without the hand that grasps it, and what can we do without the Spirit of God?"

By age 28, my life was filled with what the world offered, but I was empty inside. I was at a turning point. I could choose to turn to God or continue to reject Him. By God's grace, I repented and put my complete trust in Christ. Although far from perfect, God radically transformed and redirected my life through the power of the Holy Spirit. He can do the same for you. Acts 1:8 identifies this experience: "You shall receive power when the Holy Spirit has come upon you; and you shall be witnesses to Me...." The power of the Holy Spirit is like dynamite that ignites a hunger for

God so intense that every aspect of life is changed—we become bold, not passive; stable, not fanatical; and committed, not wavering.

Within the months that followed this experience, my passion and purpose for life became clearer than ever. I then understood Acts 3:19, "Repent therefore and be converted, that your sins may be blotted out, so that times of refreshing [revival] may come from the presence of the Lord." I truly experienced this infilling of the Spirit that is seen throughout the Scriptures (e.g., a transformed life resulting in a love for God and His Word). From this experience, came books, articles, speaking engagements, and ultimately, a church.

Like many Christians, I tend to be "safely" conservative when considering the power of the Holy Spirit; however, Scripture clearly supports the miraculous work of the Spirit today. I'm open but cautious. We need sound doctrine and the power of the Holy Spirit. As many have said before, it's possible to be "Bible taught," but not "Spirit-led"—straight as a gun barrel theologically, but just as empty. The letter kills, but the Spirit gives life (cf. 2 Corinthians 3:6).

Don't get me wrong, theological and expositional teachings are essential to Christian living, but how often are we encouraged to fast and pray as well as study? How often are we taught brokenness and repentance in addition to translating the Greek language? How often are we taught the surrendered life? We can sometimes be more concerned about having a Master's Degree than a degree from the Master.

The Holy Spirit inspired the Scriptures and empowered Jesus and the Apostles. We are desperately remiss if we fail to recognize His vital role in our lives. I agree with Leonard Ravenhill, "We need to close every church in the land for one Sunday and cease listening to a man so we can hear the groan of the Spirit which we in our lush pews have forgotten." Granted, we have gifted leaders who are led by the Spirit, but we, individually, need to spend serious time searching and listening to God.[1]

Sadly, we often pray on the run and scurry through a 5-minute devotional, yet we devote hours to television, movies, and the Internet, and we wonder why we know little of the power of the Spirit. We must spend much time seeking God if we are to continue in the power of the Holy Spirit.

⇒ If you're having difficulty succeeding so far in this forty journey, take time and ask God to strengthen you; then simply submit to the work of His Spirit.[2] That could be as simple as obeying what He has told you to do, or something more challenging such as making a major change in your life.

DAY FOURTEEN

MEN—LIFE IS A BATTLEGROUND, NOT A PLAYGROUND

A young Podcast listener once wrote, *"My dad is so self-absorbed that he doesn't notice that we are dying spiritually, relationally, and emotionally. He acts like we are an inconvenience, and he is very disrespectful to my mother. At church, he says all the right things, but at home, he's yelling, gone, or too tired to spend any time with us. I just want my dad back."*

We are in desperate need of genuine leadership—broken, humble men—men who are not afraid to admit that they need God; men who are more worried about prayer than about status and recognition; men who petition God rather than position themselves.

The state of the family today is disheartening. Men have largely forsaken their God-given role as spiritual leaders in their homes; that, no one can deny. Many know more about their favorite athletes than their wives and children. They'd rather be seen leaving a bar than leaving a church.

Men need to understand that knowing is not the same as doing. In addition to knowing God's Word, we also do it. To carry the weight of responsibility as husbands, leaders, and fathers we must obey the word of God, not just quote it; we must live it out at home rather than appear *spiritual* at church.

Unmistakably, the foundation of obedience that we build today provides the strength that weathers the storm tomorrow. Unfortunately, today's society focuses largely on external factors such as money, position, status, and recognition. These superficial values have left our nation in a moral, as well as a spiritual crisis. We've become a society focused on prosperity instead of provision; we value wealth instead of wisdom and we are drawn to charisma instead of character.

Men, you're not called to be a passive, weak, indecisive partner—you're called to protect, lead, and guard your family. You are to initiate prayer, defend your wife, shepherd your children, and make your home a holy sanctuary, not a breeding ground for Satan. You're called to fight the enemy, not flee from him. I'm tired of weak, passive men who never contend, stand, or fight for anything worth dying for.

Our nation is looking for character, our wives are looking for leaders, and our children are looking for fathers. Men, stop the silly video games, minimize time on Facebook, kill your porn habit, and tell your ungodly friends to hit the road. You're called to lead, love, and die, if necessary, for your family. We are the reason that the nation is deteriorating. We are the reason the family is breaking down. We must stop blaming everything from God to the government; we are the stench in the nostrils of a righteous, holy, and pure God.

Men, wake up! Life is a battleground, not a playground!

I can hear it now: "Shane, you're being too hard on the guys." In my opinion, just the opposite is true. Most men do not need to be encouraged and coddled; they need to be confronted and challenged . . . then they can be encouraged.

One problem in the American church is that we always encourage but rarely challenge; we cuddle but don't confront; we laugh but rarely weep. An African pastor was asked, "Why is there so much counseling in the American church but not in the African church?" He answered, "In America, you counsel. In Africa, we repent." Repentance leads to restoration. Take time now and repent if you need a spiritual reset.

⇒ How can you begin leading your family? Start by praying for them each day. Choose a few passages of scripture that can be read and discussed. Finally, do hard and challenging things that build you up spiritually. Spend quality time with your family. If single, begging to build character now, not after you're married. That rarely works.

DAY FIFTEEN

THE DIFFERENCE BETWEEN HAPPINESS AND JOY

In the years preceding my commitment to Christ, I was restless and unhappy. I thought that a move would help; therefore, I would often spend time in the mountains or at the beach, but the void never left. It would be years later before I would understand why I lacked fulfillment and a genuine passion for life.

We were designed to fellowship with God, to do His will, and to obey His principles. Living outside of this plan often brings discouragement and disappointment. Searching for purpose affects every area of life. It can determine where we'll live, whom we'll marry, where we'll work, and how we'll spend our time. Unfortunately, many search for purpose and meaning in material possessions, hobbies, and other things that do not hold eternal value. If you believe that materially successful people are happy, think again.

As I said earlier, most of us understand that money can buy the best mattress, but it can't guarantee sleep. Why do millionaires, movie stars, and top entertainers often turn to spirituality, drugs, and alcohol for the answers if success satisfies? Many discover that money, fame, and recognition are not the answers.

CEOs, presidents, and vice presidents frequently admit that they are happy when they reach production goals, but very unhappy when under budget, *largely because they measure happiness by what's happening to them*. When things go well, they're happy, when things go poorly, they're unhappy. I'm not suggesting that we shouldn't be productive, but if happiness is measured by our circumstances, it's going to be a very rough road.

God plants desire in our hearts. Without desire, we are not inclined to pursue vocations like medicine, law, professional ministry, education, construction, sales, and so on. God wants us to pursue our interests. Again, He is the one who created that desire, but our definition of prosperity often centers on financial prosperity, or what makes us comfortable.

I often hear people say *it's quality, not quantity* that counts when it comes to spending time with family members. (Often, this is just an excuse to be absent from home as much as possible.) Let's apply this thought to other areas of life and test its validity. Does a quality ten-minute workout once a week produce results? Does eating a quality meal once a week lead to better health? Does spending a few quality minutes at work lead to financial success? You can see where this is going . . . both quality and quantity matter. Try this test: invite your wife and kids to honestly share how important *time* is to them; you may be surprised at their answer.

In closing, lasting hope and joy can only come from a genuine relationship with Christ. I know that I mention this quite frequently, but I'd rather err on the side of speaking too much about finding genuine peace through Jesus Christ than too little. This is where true and lasting joy comes from.

. . .

⇒ List three practical ways that you can focus on joy over happiness. My top one is being thankful for everything that God has blessed me with, as well as speaking life into others instead of constantly being critical and negative.

DAY SIXTEEN

MONEY—SERVANT OR MASTER?

Throughout the centuries, the church has watched the pendulum swing between vows of poverty and the prosperity gospel. In times past, Christians equated oaths of poverty with deep spiritual maturity, whereas today, the *prosperity gospel* claims the opposite, teaching that wealth is a sign of God's favor. Both extremes offer a false sense of spirituality. Poverty does not necessarily enhance spirituality, and the prosperity gospel is not the real gospel. God may prosper us but that is not an indication of our spirituality. The Bible teaches us that the Lord both gives and takes away (cf. Job 1:21).

For this reason, America needs a reality check. Every day, thousands of children die in some of the poorest villages on earth; almost two in three lack access to clean water, surviving on less than $2 a day. This is extremely disheartening.

The average, low-income family in America is wealthier than millions across our globe. We often fail to realize just how blessed we are. Rather than using our resources to serve us and others, they have become our master. We fail to recognize God as the true source of blessing and abundance: "We have forgotten God, and we have vainly imagined, in the deceitfulness of our hearts, that all these blessings were produced by some superior wisdom and virtue of our own" (Abraham Lincoln).[1]

Lincoln recognized that most Americans credit themselves with their success rather than God. We either worship the god of this world or the true and living God. Jesus taught, "No one can serve two masters. Either he will hate the one and love the other, or he will be devoted to the one and despise the other. You cannot serve both God and Money" (Matthew 6:24).

During this forty-day reset, consider the following and make any necessary changes:

1. Money is a heart issue. God does not need our money. Money is a gauge that measures spiritual health. This is no doubt why Jesus taught on stewardship more than any other topic, saying, "For where your treasure is, there your heart will be also" (Matthew 6:21). 1 Timothy 6:10 says, "For the love of money is a root of all kinds of evils. It is through this craving that some have wandered away from the faith and pierced themselves with many pangs." It all starts here—the love of money is a snare that leads us further and further from God.

2. Wisdom in stewardship is foundational. One definition of stewardship notes that people who have yielded control of their finances to Christ habitually honor Him in their financial decisions and steward resources that He has provided. Budgeting resources and controlled spending is wise stewardship. Do you "need" something or do you simply "want" it? This question is at the heart of good stewardship.

3. Determine how much to give on a regular basis: "Each one must give as he has decided in his heart, not reluctantly or under compulsion, for God loves a cheerful giver" (2 Corinthians 9:7). Sadly, many use this scripture to support minimal giving when it actually promotes the opposite. From my perspective, New Testament believers aren't "required" to tithe, but they should be very generous people. Ten percent is a good number to use as a starting point in a budget. David said, "I will not give the Lord that which costs me nothing" (2 Samuel 24:24). Giving to the Lord must cost something—that is true, sacrificial giving.

4. Motive is the key: The Bible tells us about a "rich fool" who said, 'I shall say to my soul, 'My soul, you have many goods laid up for many years, be contented, eat, drink and be merry.' But God said to him, 'You fool! This very night your life will be demanded from you. Then who will get what you have prepared for yourself?' This is how it will be with anyone who stores up things for himself but is not rich toward God" (Lk. 12:19-21). Having a savings account wasn't the issue, his heart was corrupt. He was a selfish, self-centered man. God judged him for it. Had the man said, "God, I have many goods laid up for many years. What would you like me to do with these resources?" he would have been in the center of God's will. This man's attitude about his money revealed his heart. In the same way, our attitude reveals the condition of our heart: "For where your treasure is, there your heart will be also" (Matthew 6:21).

⇒ Do you agree that money can be a wonderful servant, but a terrible master? If so, are there any changes that need to be made? "For what shall it profit a man, if he shall gain the whole world, and lose his own soul?" (Mark 8:36).

DAY SEVENTEEN

EXPERIENCING GOD THROUGH HOLINESS

Of all the attributes of God described in the Bible, holiness is seen most often. Men fell down in the holy presence of God. Leaders, priests, and kings all trembled at the sheer magnitude of His holiness. The angels cry, "Holy, Holy, Holy is our God." Holiness is the key to truly understanding God, and at the heart of holiness is obedience.

Sadly, many have intellectual knowledge of God but few have heart knowledge: "Blessed are those who hunger and thirst for righteousness, for they shall be filled" (Matthew 5:6). There must be a hunger and a thirst for holiness. A quick mental run-through of our media choices, checkbooks, and calendars reveals if we are truly seeking hard after God. James 1:27 says that we are to remain "unspotted" from the world—to be free from the world's corruption. We should continually ask, "Are we 'affecting' the world, or is the world 'infecting' us?"

The *Eerdman's Dictionary of the Bible* defines holiness: "The root idea of holiness is that of 'separation' or 'withdrawal'. It is a divine quality, part of the intrinsic nature of God, but absent from a fallen world." Holiness is not simply knowing about God; knowledge and holiness do not necessarily go hand-in-hand. One can have knowledge of sin but not be repentant. Holiness does not mean that we never sin. Those who seek holiness realize just how sinful they actually are. The closer we draw to God, the clearer the picture of sin becomes.

Let's be clear here: Holiness does not lead to the forgiveness of sin. God declares the believer righteous (holy) because of Christ's sacrifice on the cross. The formula "Christ plus something equals salvation" is not biblical. We are declared right before God when we put our trust in Christ, not in our *good works*. In passages where Jesus referred to helping those in need, following Him unconditionally, and dying to self, He was not saying that we are saved because we do these things, but rather, we do these things because we are saved.

Holiness is not as much about "what" I don't do as it is about "why" I don't do it. It's safe to assume that those who live strictly by rules rather than a true relationship with Christ are not holy . . . they are religious. They may avoid certain people, places, and things but still be critical, judgmental, jealous, arrogant, and angry—"having a form of godliness." Holiness involves truly seeking God versus "playing church."

Now with that said, holiness may appear as if one is following rules (avoiding people, places, and things that hinder growth) but this avoidance is fueled by a relationship with God rather than rules. This is why sin is serious: it separates us from God; it stands in direct opposition to Him. It corrupts our character and our testimony; it prevents holiness and quenches and grieves the Spirit within.

In his book on holiness, J.C. Ryle said that we must stand guard as a soldier on enemy ground. The problem is that many love the world and have a hard time separating from it. They believe in heaven, but they don't truly long for it. They "say" that they fear God but they don't live like it. They indulge temptation rather than fight it. They enjoy sin rather than confront it. And they compromise rather than conquer. The lukewarm church disdains the heat of conviction. Holiness, to them, is outdated and old-fashioned.

Make no mistake, holiness will cost something. Ryle continues with these words about making holiness a priority, "He must count it no strange thing to be mocked, ridiculed, slandered, persecuted, and even hated. He must not be surprised to find his opinions and practices in religion despised and held up to scorn." In short, we are to do what is right, not what is popular . . . pleasing God rather than man.

In closing, be aware of partial obedience—*kind of* obeying God is not obeying Him (cf. 1 Sam. 13:5–14). I knew a person who felt that God wanted them to stop drinking coffee and alcohol. Instead of obeying, they had, in their words, "just a little coffee" in the morning and a "small amount" of alcohol in the evening. The hang-up wasn't in the amount, it was in the partial obedience. It wasn't until they finally stopped compromising that God met them in a powerful and profound way. *God doesn't say, "Let's make a deal"; He says, "This is the deal".*

⇒ How about you? Are there any areas that you have not fully surrendered? Drawing a line can be out of step with the mainstream, but, like Joshua who I quoted earlier, we too must say: Choose this day whom you will serve, as for me and my house we will serve the Lord (Joshua 24:15).

DAY EIGHTEEN

IS THE WORLD INFECTING YOU?

Years ago, a Governor in the South was asked by his daughter if she could wear a certain outfit. The attire was trendy and fashionable but lacked modesty. When her request was denied, she answered back, "But everyone is wearing this style!" His answer, "You do not follow the styles, you set them."

The Christian life is a close parallel in many respects. James 1:27 says that Christians are to remain "unspotted" from the world—which literally means to be free from the world's corruption. We should continually ask, "Are we 'affecting' the world, or is the world 'infecting' us?"

How is one to be "in the world" yet not "of the world"? We are "in the world" because we live here; we cannot change that. But "of the world" means something completely different. It means to take on the world's mindset—to think and act like the culture, and often, like the media.

There is a very troubling trend toward embracing the world in the evangelical church; just look at our entertainment and lifestyle choices. Most are deeply infected by the world, and therefore, they are not truly affecting the world. Instead of acknowledging our obvious falling away from God's standard of holiness, we often excuse our actions under the guise of *relating* to the culture.

Our primary calling is not to relate to the world—it's to please God. Granted, if we fail to relate to our culture, the church can become ineffective. But when holiness is sacrificed for the sake of relating to the culture, as we see today, our relationship with God suffers. The problem isn't that we raise our standard of holiness and miss it, it's that we lower it and hit it. "Where does Christianity destroy itself in a given generation? It destroys itself by not living in the light, by professing a truth it does not obey" (A.W. Tozer).

I'm aware that I'm really driving this point home in this book, but we must be vigilant in this area if we are to truly influence and impact our culture. I'm not talking about issues such as public or private schooling, or only working for "Christian" employees; I'm defining separation as it relates to morality and behavior. This type of separation is absolutely essential when it comes to walking closely with God and resting in Him.

In short, holiness (with the right heart) is an important pillar when it comes to experiencing a spiritual reset. "All the water in the world, however hard it tried, could never sink the smallest ship unless it gets inside. And all the evil in the world, the blackest kind of sin, can never hurt you in the least unless you let it in."[1]

Second Corinthians 6:14 sheds more light on this issue, "Do not be unequally yoked together with unbelievers. For what fellowship has righteousness with lawlessness? And what communion has light with darkness?"

A yoke was a heavy harness placed on the neck of oxen as they stood side by side. The yoke was then connected to whatever was to be pulled. The oxen were much more effective and stronger as they pulled the load in unison. If one of them turned in another direction, the yoke could break or the load could tip. In the same way, unequally yoked relationships can hinder our relationship with the Lord and the direction that He wants to take us.

In addition to the partnerships mentioned above, our friendships should honor God as well. Please understand that I am not suggesting that Christians only interact with other Christians. We are called to minister to others in all areas of life. We cannot totally separate from the culture. What good is salt if it's left in the shaker? But if the friendship is pulling you in the wrong direction, it's time to re-evaluate the relationship. Hebrews 12:1 tells us to remove every weight and burden that slows us down. Negative relationships are both a weight and a burden.

If you're questioning God's existence, experiencing violent bursts of anger and rage, severely struggling with an addiction or lust, or continually feeling depressed or discouraged, evaluate your mental diet of television, movies, the Internet, music, and friends. Are they lifting you up, or pulling you down? There is no middle ground—you're being influenced one way or the other.

⇒ I've discussed this quite a bit so far, but that's because it's so important. Our mental diet affects our spiritual health. Are there any changes that need to be made in your life? If so, why wait? Get started today.

DAY NINETEEN

GOD'S WILL IS ALWAYS RIGHT ON TIME

"With the Lord one day is as a thousand years, and a thousand years as one day" (2 Peter 3:8). Although this Scripture may not apply directly to God's will, the principle still applies: His will is revealed in His time.

Granted, there are times when the Holy Spirit directs us instantly—prompting a phone call to a friend in need, or leading us to make a quick decision, but when it comes to the big picture, we sometimes only see portions of it. God often leads us through one open door at a time. "When God calls me, he makes it possible for me to move in the direction he is leading" (J.I. Packer).

For example, when I felt a deep conviction to leave an eight-year profession, I only saw glimpses of the big picture. Although it seemed very unlikely at the time, I saw myself writing books and speaking. I had no idea how it would all unfold, but I knew that I needed to have faith and trust God no matter how long it took. God began to open doors, and I walked through.

Additionally, I had peace. In the same way, you may not know exactly what you are going to do with your life, but God does. Be patient . . . God may lead more by withholding information than by supplying it. This can help us stay focused on the task at hand, remain obedient, and walk by faith. For example, had I known that I was going to encounter a few years of financial hardship and dig ditches for a living when I stepped away from a six-figure income, I might not have left. I only saw glimpses of His will for a reason: He wanted me to pay attention to where I was as well as where I was going. Enjoy each and every day, and don't be in a hurry—especially when raising young children.

As you wait on God, don't be surprised by challenges: "We are hard-pressed on every side, yet not crushed; we are perplexed, but not in despair" (2 Corinthians 4:8). When we are walking according to God's will, the struggles that we encounter are not necessarily an indicator that we are out of God's will; He may be molding us, or they may be part of an unfolding plan. God often directs us by removing us from our comfort zone. He closes one door but opens another.

God strengthens and prepares us so that we can handle the weight of what He has called us to do. Figuratively speaking, you don't see a young apple tree bear abundant fruit; the tree would collapse under the weight. We also have growing to do. There are personality issues, attitudes, and certain habits that may need to be adjusted. There is a saying in the construction business that "the deeper the foundation, the stronger the structure." The depth of our spiritual foundation also determines how much we can carry. Don't be frustrated; God may be building and strengthening your foundation, and aligning your will with His.

I once believed that life was easy in the center of God's will, and if it wasn't easy, then I was out of His will. This isn't necessarily true. Yes, we should have peace in the center of God's will, but not freedom from difficult circumstances. At times, we may fight bouts of anxiety, depression, and fear. Many biblical heroes fought hardship and anxiety while being in the center of God's will. How can we determine if a challenge is a result of being in God's will, or because of disobedience? First, ask yourself if your motives are pure and honest. Second, focus on obeying God's Word and the convictions of the Holy Spirit. Third, seek biblical counsel and use wisdom. He will direct you one way or the other.

Again, try to see challenges as opportunities for growth. Being in the center of God's will does not prevent challenges; it sometimes creates them. In Matthew 7:24-27, Jesus tells the story of a wise man who built his house on solid rock (God's Word), rather than on shifting sand (man's philosophy). As a result, his house withstood the storm, but the foolish man who built his house on sand lost everything.

⇒ Remember, both men encountered the storm. Adversity comes to all of us. How can you better prepare for storms and weather them successfully? I've found that trusting in God's sovereignty helps a great deal.

DAY TWENTY

THE COST OF SPEAKING THE TRUTH

There is a cost to speaking the truth. This realization came many years ago when I was asked to speak at the annual conference for the American Baptists, unaware that they were about to divide over an important biblical issue.

Within minutes of beginning my message, a few people began to leave the large auditorium. Although it was clear that I had struck a nerve, the clearest message came when a woman approached the platform and attempted to disrupt the service. I told her that I would be happy to talk with her after the service.

Afterward, a large line of people waited to talk to me. I will never forget the very angry 12-year old girl. My heart sank when she said, "I hate everything you had to say. It was mean and hateful!" Though shocked by her comment, I was moved with compassion for such a young life filled with passion for the wrong things. Others asked if I ever received death threats.

As I boarded the plane, I was perplexed and confused. I prayed, "Lord, what's wrong. I'm simply speaking Your Word and genuinely loving these people." The words of Titus Brandsma (martyred at Dachau under Hitler) began to ring true, "Those who want to win the world for Christ must have the courage to come into conflict with it."

I buckled my seat, anxious to head for the familiar comfort of home, but I knew that my life had made a turn. This gospel of love had, ironically, become a message of hate to those who oppose it: "A time is coming when anyone who kills you will think he is offering a service to God" (John 16:2).

Speaking the truth was going to cost me (and it will cost you). I knew that my kids would someday be old enough to ask about the reason behind the hate mail, mean remarks, and indignant looks. While most feedback is very encouraging, those who are upset will often stop at nothing to get their point across. Do I enjoy this? That goes without an answer. Although many applaud my boldness, if the truth be told, my life would be much easier if I took a secular job and avoided controversy. But I cannot. God radically changed my life by the power of His Spirit through His truth: "It's like a fire in my bones! I am worn out trying to hold it in! I can't do it!" (Jeremiah 20:9).

The only difference between believers and unbelievers is that believers are simply forgiven—they have embraced God's gracious gift of forgiveness, wholeness, and restoration through Christ's sacrifice on the cross. Because of the cross, sin has been conquered and atoned for (cf. Romans 6). "If you confess with your mouth the Lord Jesus and believe in your heart that God has raised Him from the dead, you will be saved" (Romans 10:9).

My goal is to simply share God's gracious gift. If being labeled narrow-minded, legalistic, judgmental, arrogant, and intolerant is the cost of speaking the truth in love, so be it. In 2 Timothy 4:1-2, Paul instructs Timothy, "I solemnly charge you in the presence of

God and of Christ Jesus, who is to judge the living and the dead, and by His appearing and His kingdom: preach the word; be ready in season and out of season; reprove, rebuke, exhort, with great patience and instruction."

Paul is saying to preach the difficult truths as well as the joyful ones; preach the cross and the new life; preach hell and preach heaven; preach damnation and preach salvation; preach sin and preach grace; preach wrath and preach love; preach judgment and preach mercy; preach obedience and preach forgiveness; preach "God "is love" but don't forget that God is just. It is the love of God that compels us to share all of His truth.

⇒ In what ways are you prepared to speak the truth? Why do you think that people are often afraid to share the truth? What is one way that you can share the truth today?

DAY TWENTY-ONE

I'M TOO BUSY TO PRAY

The one thing that all great Christian men and women have is the one thing that many others lack—a powerful prayer life. Great Christians are known as men and women of extraordinary prayer, brokenness, and humility, filled and clothed with power from on high. *The men and women who do the most for God are always men and women of prayer.* "Prayer is not a preparation for the battle; it is the battle" (Leonard Ravenhill).

Here are a few examples from the past to motivate you during the last half of this forty-day reset: E.M. Bounds, who was born in 1835, began his three-hour prayer routine at 4 am. To him, prayer was not a prelude; it was a priority. Edward Payson, who ministered during the Second Great Awakening, was said to have worn grooves into his hardwood floors as a result of prayer. It was said of John Hyde who left for the mission field in 1892 that he would stay on his face before God until the answer came. William Bramwell, a powerful Methodist circuit rider, often spent hours a day on his knees until his death in 1818.

Adoniram Judson attributed his success as a missionary in Burma to a life of prayer, as did J. Hudson Taylor, founder of the China Inland Mission. George Mueller, who never asked for a dime, petitioned God for millions of dollars to fund his orphanages in the 1800s. It was not uncommon for the great Scottish preacher, John Welch, who died in 1622, to spend four to six hours in prayer. John Fletcher, one of the leaders of the Methodist movement, "stained the walls of his room with the breath of his prayers" until his death in 1785.

At this point, many will say, "Wait a minute. Who has that much time to pray; we're all too busy." You're right, but let me be frank: If we're too busy to cultivate a prayer life that places God first—we're too busy. We should never allow our relationship with Him to suffer because we're too busy. "We must spend much time on our knees before God if we are to continue in the power of the Holy Spirit" (R.A. Torrey).

If you truly want to build intimacy with God, you'll have to remove less important things from your life. Years ago, I realized that if I wanted to grow spiritually, some things would have to go, or, at the very least, be minimized; I needed to reprioritize my life. Instead of watching hours of television a day, I began to devote my time to activities that strengthened my relationship with the Lord. I cannot begin to tell you how much of a difference that made. Although far from perfect, I began to put first things first. As a result, I began to hunger for God's Word and spiritual truth like never before. It's impossible to develop a deep respect and desire for God if we repeatedly fill our minds with things that oppose Him.

The depth of your relationship with God is in direct proportion to the depth of your commitment to Him; great commitment, great relationship; poor commitment, poor relationship. Prayer matters: it equips, anoints, and empowers. God-given authority and prayer go hand-in-hand. You can't have one without the other.

⇒ Put prayer and fasting on your calendar and begin today. "Prayer is reaching out after the unseen; fasting is letting go of all that is seen and temporal. Fasting helps express, deepen, confirm the resolution that we are ready to sacrifice anything, even ourselves to attain what we seek for the kingdom of God" (Andrew Murray).

DAY TWENTY-TWO

AVOID THESE THREE DESTRUCTIVE INFLUENCES

Speaking from personal experience and observation, I have witnessed many sabotage their lives through three destructive forces. Although I have touched on these throughout the book, I wanted to lay all three out in one reflection. According to 1 John 2:16, they are: the lust of the flesh (what we crave), the lust of the eyes (what is pleasing to the eye), and the pride of life (arrogance).

1. **The lust of the flesh.** Lust can be defined as an uncontrolled or intense desire that crosses the boundary lines into sin. Although the most common meaning relates to strong sexual desire, it can also apply to any type of intense desire. All of us struggle with lust in some form or another. The question is, do we entertain the thought until it fuels desire and brings forth sin, or do we walk away? Desire is not wrong, but what we do with it can be. If our hearts are sincere and teachable, God can bless us, but if we purposely engage in sin, we remove His protection. Being tempted isn't sin—surrendering to it is. God is merciful to forgive and bestow blessings as we repent and make necessary lifestyle changes.

Feelings of lust can be overcome when we read His Word, shield our eyes and ears from the things that tempt us, educate ourselves, apply wisdom, and surround ourselves with those who lift us up rather than pull us down. Addictions can also be classified as the lust of the flesh. Addiction often means giving oneself up to a habit and then becoming dependent upon that habit. There are many different things that people can become addicted to, but usually the lust of the flesh is at the root of the addiction.

2. **The lust of the eyes** can be defined as coveting, or desiring something such as a trophy wife, an expensive home or vehicle, or other things that symbolize money and possessions. Workaholics, for example, can appear as hard-working and industrious, but their focus on their work eventually robs them of other relationships, and the spiritual and emotional health of their family is neglected. Many men in America will accept difficult employees, face challenging situations on the job, work exhausting hours, commit fully to the cause of the company and do whatever it takes to get the job done, yet, unfortunately, they severely neglect a marriage—sometimes it appears as if they'd rather lose a wife than a career.

When we fall prey to the lust of the eyes, our focus often shifts from Christ-centered to self-centered. The next time a decision needs to be made, try asking, "Will this decision please God?" In Matthew 4:8-9 Jesus was also tempted by the lust of the eyes. It states, "The devil took Him to a very high mountain and showed Him all the kingdoms of the world and their glory; and he said to Him, 'All these things I will give You, if You fall down and worship me'." Jesus rejected the devil's proposal and defeated him with the Word of God, saying: "For it is written, 'You shall worship the Lord your God, and serve Him only'" (Matthew

4:10). In the same way, we have the Word of God available to us. Don't become frustrated—change takes time. The process requires patience, consistency, and obedience in doing what is right.

3. **The pride of life** is the opposite of humility. It can be defined as conceit, or a sense of superiority in who we are or what we have. Proverbs 6:16-17 says, "The Lord hates a proud look.." Self-centeredness is closely related to pride. When we believe that our needs are more important than the needs of others, and we think more highly of ourselves than we should, pride is a problem and it will severely hinder our progress.

Pride is the only disease known to man that makes everybody sick except the person who has it. A popular saying bears consideration—God intended that we love people and use things; instead, we tend to love things and use people. Pride causes us to take pleasure in the things of the world rather than the things of God. Husbands and wives don't marry filled with love and passion one day only to lose it the next. Marriage slowly deteriorates through more attention to self than spouse. Most who are divorced will say that their marriage was initially good, but with time, one or both stopped loving—largely because of selfishness.

⇒ If the enemy "goes to and fro like a roaring lion seeking whom he may devour" (1 Peter 5:8), and "the eyes of the Lord run to and fro throughout the whole earth, to show Himself strong on behalf of those whose heart is loyal to Him," (2 Chronicles 16:9); who finds you—the adversary, or God? Are you loyal to God by obeying His Word, or do you often stray from the Shepherd and become easy prey because of pride and disobedience?

DAY TWENTY-THREE

THE SINFUL NATURE IS AT WAR WITH GOD

A young man, determined to find help for his troubled life, walked to a neighboring church. He told the pastor that his life was meaningless and in constant turmoil. He wanted to make better choices, but couldn't.

He described the conflict: "It's as if I have two dogs constantly battling within me. One dog is evil, while the other is good. The battles are long and difficult; they drain me emotionally and mentally." Without a moment's thought, the pastor asked, "Which dog wins the battles?" Hesitantly, the young man admitted, "The evil dog." The pastor looked at him and said, "That's the one you feed the most. You need to starve that dog to death!"

The pastor realized, as should we, that the source of our strength comes from the food that we choose. What we feed grows, and what grows becomes the dominating force within our lives. Sin never stands still—it either grows or withers depending on whether you feed or starve it. Which dog wins the battle in your mind?

Galatians 5:17 says that the Spirit gives us desires that are opposite from what our sinful nature desires, and that these two forces are constantly fighting against each other. As a result, our choices are rarely free from this conflict. Don't be alarmed. The fact that there is a fight confirms the value of our commitment.

The door of temptation swings both ways—you can enter or exit. That's why we need to be very selective in what we watch and listen to, and how we spend our time. Why would we willingly walk into the enemy's camp? Why would we feed wrong desires and thoughts? Feeding the flesh does nothing but bring war against the spirit.

If we could clearly see where sin was leading, most of us would reconsider our options. The enemy blinds us to the consequences of sin and entices us with its pleasures. If one could see that one, "harmless" little sexual sin, drink, or hit would lead to adultery, divorce, separation from children, depression, and despair, he or she would probably change the behavior in a heartbeat. We're often too smart to take large, deliberate plunges off the cliff, but we can be enticed to take one step at a time, one compromise at a time, one sin at a time—until it's too late!

Proverbs 23:7 says that as a man thinks in his heart, so is he. And Jesus said that the lamp of the body is the eye. When your eye is good your body will be full of light. When your eye is bad your body will be full of darkness. (Refer to Luke 11:34.) Our thoughts become words, our words become actions, our actions become habits. Who is shaping your thoughts? A daily diet of violence, lust, anger, and depression will fuel those very things in your life. This isn't rocket science: are you viewing darkness or reading God's Light (His Word)? Are you watching horror movies or praying and fasting for America? Are you watching

HBO and Netflix, or watching shows that are true, noble, and upright (cf. Philippians 4:8)?

One of the reasons why men and women struggle with sin more than they should is because they feed it throughout the day. It's difficult to avoid dangerous, sinful emotions while continually watching movies and TV programs that promote them. As a matter of fact, many cases of sexual violence can be traced directly back to pornography. Yes, I have been talking about this quite a bit. But the more I pastor a church the more I realize: *What we embrace eventually embraces us.*

Too many sermons these days only focus on positives. A pastor actually told me that he doesn't get specific on these types of things. He added, "It's the Holy Spirit's job to convict, not mine." But it's our job as preachers to convict people with the Word as the Holy Spirit works in their hearts. Leonard Ravenhill once said, "There are only two kinds of persons: those dead in sin and those dead to sin." If people are never convicted by the Word or from the pulpit, how will they ever turn from their sin?

Don't let all this discourage you, "Greater is He who is in you than he who is in the world" (1 John 4:4). The key is to maintain your loyalty to Christ and to be pure vessels that He can use. "For though we walk in the flesh, we do not war according to the flesh. For the weapons of our warfare are not carnal but mighty in God for pulling down strongholds, casting down arguments and every high thing that exalts itself against the knowledge of God, bringing every thought into captivity to the obedience of Christ" (2 Corinthians 10:3-5).

⇒ Paul understood, as should we, that the battlefield is the mind: Good thoughts will eventually produce good actions. Begin here and fall forward into God's arms of restoration and forgiveness. In what areas can you begin focusing on the things of God instead of negative, godless media?

DAY TWENTY-FOUR

UNDERSTANDING TEMPTATION

Alexander was trying to save his pennies so he could buy a baseball bat. But he had a hard struggle. One night when he was saying his prayers, his mother heard him say fervently, "O Lord, please help me save my money for a baseball bat. And, God, don't let the ice cream man come down this street anymore!"

Isn't that true of temptation? It takes from us, while at the same time, it looks so appealing. Theologian Klyne Snodgrass states it well, "Mention of the 'schemes' of the devil reminds us of the trickery by which evil and temptation present themselves in our lives. Evil rarely looks evil until it accomplishes its goal; it gains entrance by appearing attractive, desirable, and perfectly legitimate. It is a baited and camouflaged trap."

That's important to note: *we often miss evil for what it really is until after it has accomplished its purpose.* Only by comparing our thoughts and actions to God's Word can we have the insight to see beyond the circumstances. Temptation is also an opportunity to do what is right by turning from it. 1 Corinthians 10:13 states, "No temptation has overtaken you except such as is common to man; but God is faithful, who will not allow you to be tempted beyond what you are able, but with the temptation will also make the way of escape, that you may be able to bear it." Again, the door of temptation swings both ways. If we choose to enter, once inside, we may not see the exit sign so clearly again.

Consider these points:

1. The flesh is in rebellion against God. Puritan author, John Owen, writes, "Secret lusts lie lurking in your own heart which will never give up until they are either destroyed or satisfied." The flesh—although it feels comfortable and natural at times—is not a friend to be trusted: "The carnal mind is enmity against God" (Romans 8:7). Enmity is not just an enemy; an enemy can be reconciled, but enmity is in direct opposition to the will of God. In short, the flesh says, "Feed me so I can destroy you ... destroy your health, your relationships, your soul." C.H. Spurgeon warned, "Beware of no man more than of yourself; we carry our worst enemies within us."

2. The devil doesn't make us do anything, he simply presents the bait. For example, the devil doesn't show a young couple the pain and anguish and the years of regret that premarital sex brings; he deceives them with temporary enjoyment and a false sense of freedom from responsibility. He has been deceiving since the beginning of time. Although the enemy will come against our family and our finances, we cannot blame him; we must take responsibility for our own poor choices when warranted.

3. Be aware of "opportune times." Recall Luke 4:13, "And when the devil had ended every temptation, he departed from him until an opportune time." In battle, the enemy attacks at opportune times. "Opportune times" in the Greek language is like a favorable wind blowing a ship toward its destination. Again, 1 John 2:16 reminds us that the world entices through cravings for physical pleasure and through covetousness, and through pride in our achievements and possessions. These are the three areas where the enemy will concentrate his focus. Be aware of these "opportune times."

4. The source of our strength comes from the food that we choose. What we feed grows, and what grows becomes the strong and dominating force within our lives. Sin never stands still—it either grows or withers depending on whether we feed or starve it. Our thoughts become words, our words become actions, our actions become habits. Who is shaping your thoughts? A daily diet of violence, lust, anger, and depression will fuel those very things in your life.

Again, the devil doesn't make us do anything; he simply presents the bait. James 1:14-15 says that each one of us "is tempted when, by his own evil desire, he is dragged away and enticed. Then, after desire has conceived, it gives birth to sin; and sin, when it is full-grown, gives birth to death (e.g. feed me so I can destroy you)."

⇒ Be encouraged: When you truly seek God's help, you can control temptation instead of allowing temptation to control you. The key is to pray for strength and wisdom, and to be mindful of the weapons of warfare (see Ephesians 6). An immediate exit at the first sign of temptation will encourage victory. Turn back from temptation today.

DAY TWENTY-FIVE

HOPE FOR THE HURTING

No doubt many reading this book are going through (or have gone through) a difficult marriage. For this reason, I want to offer hope in today's *reflection*. If you are single, you'll need this information as well, so keep reading.

In the book, *Sacred Thirst*, the author writes, "The bride and groom are standing in front of everyone, looking better than they are ever going to look again, getting so much attention and affirmation. Everybody even stands when they walk in so it's easy to think this marriage, at least, is about them. It's not. Just look at the worn-out parents sitting in the first pew—they understand this. The only reason these parents are still married is because long ago they learned how to handle the hurt they caused each other. They know that the last thing you ever want to do with hurt is to let it define you."

This last statement offers one of the most profound points that I've read on brokenness. Those who do not allow hurt to entrap them can turn brokenness into an unbreakable force, but those shackled by past pain are truly imprisoned by it. Married or divorced, the walls we build to protect may eventually imprison.

How can we undo the emotional pain that we experience from failed relationships? First, we must understand that our mind is where battles are either won or lost. Those who do not forgive or release bitterness, anger, and hurt, never experience freedom, happiness, or 'true' restoration. It all starts here.

Ephesians 4:31-32 says, "Let all bitterness, wrath, anger, clamor, and evil speaking be put away from you, with all malice. And be kind to one another, tenderhearted, forgiving one another, even as God in Christ forgave you." Simply stated, if you fail to forgive, then bitterness and anger, though skillfully masked, can and will tarnish your relationships.

Regardless of what you have endured, God can deliver you from the emotional scars and feelings of abandonment, and break the walls that imprison you. God can turn brokenness into an unbreakable force, but it is imperative that your mind is renewed by applying biblical principles, beginning with forgiveness.

Those who have walked in true forgiveness know that God restores. It's been well stated that life makes us bitter or it makes us better—the choice is ours. God can deliver those broken by a failed marriage, but for change to occur on the outside (i.e., remarriage or restoration) it first must occur on the inside. Strongholds include bitterness, pride, lust, selfishness, substance abuse, toxic relationships, anger, and physical abuse, to name a few. These destructive influences hinder the healing and rebuilding process. Healing begins with a commitment to work on those areas known to be detrimental to your spiritual health and the health of the relationship.

Do you desire peace and joy again? Simply return to God: "You will seek Me and find Me when you search for Me with all your heart" (Jeremiah 29:13). Full surrender provides fertile ground for joy and peace.

Don't allow past brokenness to cause future pain. Regret and failure will linger as long as we let them. Scripture is very clear: We are to forget those things that are behind us and focus on those things ahead. You can't change where you've been, but you can change where you're going.

I learned that shepherds, from time to time, broke the leg of a lamb that continually wandered from the flock and, thus, the shepherd's protection. The shepherd would then splint the broken leg and carry the lamb on his shoulders for weeks until the leg healed. As painful as this was for the lamb, it was necessary to protect it from being ravished by wolves or other predators.

In time, through the broken and dependent relationship, the lamb learned to walk and to remain in the protective presence of his shepherd. This concept was well stated by David in Psalms 51:8, "That the bones You have broken may rejoice." And Isaiah reminds us, "All we like sheep have gone astray" (53:6). Ironically, many thank the Lord for using their divorce to bring them back to the Good Shepherd.

⇒ What will it take to bring you back? A deliberate decision to stay close to Him can avoid unneeded pain and provide safety and protection.

DAY TWENTY-SIX

UNDERSTANDING GRACE

"Do not think that I came to destroy the Law or the Prophets. I did not come to destroy but to fulfill. For assuredly, I say to you, till heaven and earth pass away, one jot or one tittle will by no means pass from the law till all is fulfilled..." (Matthew 5:17-20).

Some says that because we are "no longer under law, but under grace" (Romans 6:14) that the "thou shalt nots" no longer apply. But this twisting of the truth attempts to justify sin. "The moment you begin to question the authority of the Old Testament, you are, of necessity, questioning the authority of the Son of God!" (D. Martyn Lloyd-Jones).[1]

In Matthew 5, Jesus clarifies His ultimate authority. And because the Jews often wrongly viewed Christianity as a replacement of the law rather than a fulfillment, Jesus clears this fallacy by stating, "I did not come to destroy but to fulfill." This statement set the tone for the rest of the conversation, namely, Jesus' teachings are in complete harmony with the Old Testament. Granted, the ceremonial and dietary laws of the Old Testament do not apply today, but the "moral" laws (kill, steal, lie, adultery, bear false witness, etc.) are as significant today as they have been throughout history.

The legal consequences of wrong actions may have changed, but the moral implications remain the same. For instance, even though we no longer stone to death those who commit adultery, this does not mean that adultery is acceptable or any less dangerous. Adultery is morally wrong even though there aren't legal consequences.

When it comes to the Old Testament Law, wisdom avoids holding to one of two extremes: Always quoting the Law, or always saying, "We're not under the Law." Both truths are essential: The law was given by Moses, but grace and truth came by Jesus Christ. The law and grace are married, rather than divorced. Galatians 3:19 says that the law was given alongside the promise of the Messiah, to show people their sins.

The Apostle Paul presents the question, "Is there a conflict, then, between God's law and God's promises?" Absolutely not! If the law could save us then we could be made right with God by obeying it. But the Scriptures declare that we are prisoners of sin. We receive God's promise of freedom only by believing in Jesus Christ (cf. Galatians 3:21-23). Before the perfect sacrifice of Christ was available, all were placed under guard by the law. *The law condemns, Christ releases.*

Again, this doesn't mean that God's moral standards are to be dismissed. Quite the contrary, grace does not relieve us of responsibility; we now live under a higher standard when grace, not rules, guides our decisions. We who are living under grace should not want to continue in sin.

In the Old Testament, the covering for sin was found in the sacrificial system: "without the shedding of blood there is no forgiveness of sin." But in the New Testament, Christ's perfect sacrifice (His fulfillment of the law through a blood sacrifice), is now the redeeming factor: "God made Him who had no sin to be sin for us, so that in Him we might become the righteousness of God" (2 Corinthians 5:21).

You may say, "But I'm a good person." Good according to whose standard? Good wasn't good enough for Noah, Abraham, Moses, David, Peter, Paul, and John, and it's not good enough for you. The cross isn't just another symbol or a charm to ward off evil; it wasn't intended to be displayed as décor. Christ bore, endured, and received the full force of God's wrath on the cross. The full penalty of the law was paid in full. Again, the law condemns but Christ releases.

⇒ Have you repented from your sin, confessed Christ as Lord and Savior, and embraced His perfect sacrifice? Life often ends before we are ready. Are you ready? You don't want to live with a question mark here.

DAY TWENTY-SEVEN

A WORD TO THE CRITICAL HEART

In last week's reflection, I mentioned that popular opinion says that because we are "no longer under law, but under grace" (Romans 6:14). Some even say that the "thou shalt nots" don't really apply today. Granted, we cannot separate the letter of the law from the spirit of grace; they are inseparable. Legalists, however, vocalize God's wrath, judgment, and condemnation, but avoid mentioning His love, grace, and forgiveness. Conviction that is not undergirded by love harms the true gospel.

In Matthew 5:21-22, Jesus said, "You have heard that it was said to those of old, 'You shall not murder, and whoever murders will be in danger of the judgment.' But I say to you that whoever is angry with his brother without a cause shall be in danger of the judgment." He went straight to the issue and condemned the critical, judgmental heart.

Today we might judge others in regard to women wearing head coverings, homeschooling, alcohol, sabbaths, festivals, entertainment, make-up, certain translations of the Bible, attire, fasting perfectly, and so on. For example, a legalist might say that salvation is dependent on such things as keeping the Sabbath or celebrating the Jewish festivals.

Is it wise to take a day of rest and honor God? Can people still celebrate the festivals and benefit from their observance? Absolutely, but they are not tied to salvation. The New Testament tells us not to let others judge us in connection with the festivals or sabbaths, or for us to judge them (cf. Colossians 2:16). The underlying attitude of legalism is arrogant and hyper-spiritual. I've even had a few people tell me I'm not a real pastor because I don't wear a suit and tie, and have never been to seminary. Although education is vital, I'm more concerned about having a degree from the Master than a Master's Degree. Leonard Ravenhill often said, "You can have thirty-two degrees and still be frozen [cold to the things of God]."

Legalism also says, "Unless you belong to 'our' church and are baptized here, we can't assure you of salvation." Is church membership wise and baptism important? Absolutely, but salvation is not contingent upon them. We are in error any time we add something to Christ's finished work on the cross. Actions should stem from a heart of love and grace ("the spirit of the law") and not as a legalistic expression that can lead to bondage ("the letter of the law").

Most of Galatians was written because early believers added rules to grace, "You foolish Galatians! Who has bewitched you? Before your very eyes Jesus Christ was clearly portrayed as crucified. I would like to learn just one thing from you: Did you receive the Spirit by the works of the law, or by believing what you heard? Are you so foolish? After beginning by means of the Spirit, are you now trying to finish by means of the flesh?" (3:1-3).

. . .

⇒ Are you an overbearing and legalistic Christian, or are you an "anything goes under grace" liberal Christian? In any case, in order to walk in love and holiness and grace and purity, you may need to repent of destructive attitudes. We've all been guilty of either extreme, myself included. Repentance releases the shackles of bondage from either extreme.

DAY TWENTY-EIGHT

PRONE TO WANDER - LORD I FEEL IT

"Prone to wander, Lord, I feel it, prone to leave the God I love." Written in 1757, these lyrics echo with great clarity to a generation that has wandered so far off that we can barely hear God's call to return to Him.

Wander means to depart, stray, or retreat from what we know to be right. As a result, guilt and shame can dominate our lives. Proverbs 13:15 reminds us that "the way of the transgressor" is hard. For many, this is an understatement if we are fighting against God... fighting against what we know to be right.

In the same way that the DMV offers a certificate of non-operation when a vehicle is not working properly, wandering from God makes us ineffective, unproductive, negative, angry, depressed, disgruntled, discouraged, critical, and lifeless. It's clear from Scripture that the wanderer within must be restrained, but how do we restrain a nature prone to wander?

First John 1:9 offers the first glimpse of hope, "If we confess our sins, he is faithful and just to forgive us our sins and to cleanse us from all unrighteousness." Acts 3:19 adds that repentance leads to times of refreshing. Repentance and obedience to God's Word frees us from shame and guilt, and gets us back on track. Honest self-examination of our heart must take place.

1 Samuel 15:23 adds, "For rebellion is like the sin of divination, and arrogance like the evil of idolatry." God is not saying that He will reject a Christian when they rebel (or we'd all be in trouble); He is saying that disobedience is the same as magic and divination. At the heart of magic is rebellion; at the heart of false worship is self-exaltation. There is a deeper anointing, a more powerful place of worship, a more prominent place of service that flows from obedience. When "we reject the word of the Lord" through disobedience there is a high price to pay.

Pride blinds us spiritually, as illustrated in the life of the famous boxer Muhammad Ali. As the story goes, Ali was asked by a flight attendant to put on his seat belt before the plane took off. He shot back, "Superman don't need no seat belt." To that, she replied, "Superman don't need no airplane." Obadiah 1:3 says, "The pride of your heart has deceived you." The Lord detests the proud in heart. You can be sure of this: They will not go unpunished (cf. Proverbs 16:5). But keep reading, there is encouragement.

Often, it is the father who wanders first because the enemy is relentless and goes after those who are called to lead. "Today, virtually every societal problem, social injustice and behavioral abnormality can be traced back to absent, delinquent, misbehaving, drunk, or sexually immoral dads who didn't respect or understand their enormous calling" (Kenny Luck).

Kenny continues, "Girls often find themselves mistreated, miscast, misused, and undervalued. What they need is guidance, esteem, honor and worth that only a father can give. Same goes for boys. They just have a different set of statistics. Men are appointed by God to make our children secure. God's highest calling for man is to be a husband or father."

⇒ In the depths of a despairing world, we cannot forget about God's grace and love. You may feel that you've done too much damage, but don't lose heart. You'll be amazed at what God can do with humility, brokenness, and repentance. You may not be able to change your circumstances immediately, but God can change your heart from a wanderer to a worshiper and reposition you back into the center of His will. It's not too late! Ask Him to do this today.

DAY TWENTY-NINE

THE CURE FOR DOUBT AND FEAR

"Now it came to pass, when Jesus finished commanding His twelve disciples, that He departed from there to teach and to preach in their cities. And when John had heard in prison about the works of Christ, he sent two of his disciples and said to Him, 'Are You the Coming One, or do we look for another'?" (Matthew 11:1-3).

Imagine the scene above. John the Baptist, this mighty man of God, was now in prison. He may be thinking, "Why am I here? I'm doing God's will. My life is not going like I planned!"

Like John, it's okay to ask God about our doubts and fears if we are sincere and genuine. God says, "Come, let us reason together" (Isaiah 1:8), and "He who asks for wisdom" will receive it (James 1:5). But if doubt turns us away from God, serious readjustments need to be made.

The devil used doubt to mislead Eve, "Did God really say?" (cf. Genesis 3). Any time we question God's truth with a sarcastic and arrogant attitude, there will be ramifications. But if we approach Him with a sincere heart, a heart that is humble and teachable, He will lead us in the right direction.

Granted, some questions will not be answered on this side of heaven. For example, although I don't question God's perfect justice, I don't fully comprehend hell and eternal separation, or some of the events in the Old Testament. My finite mind cannot grasp the full picture. But I'm not going to doubt God over a mystery.

Matthew 11 continues, "Jesus answered and said to them, 'Go and tell John the things which you hear and see: the blind see and the lame walk; the lepers are cleansed and the deaf hear; the dead are raised up and the the poor have the gospel preached to them" (Matthew 11:4-5). Talk about fruit!

Fruit reveals what seeds were planted, and wise decisions can be seen in what is produced: "wisdom is justified by her children" (cf. Matt. 11:19). The fruit of genuine Christianity is amazing: from individual to large scale social change, from changed lives to bondages being broken, from building hospitals and schools and missions, from helping the poor and the dying, even to the giving of oneself for the truth of God's Word, Christianity has influenced large-scale changes because it first transformed the hearts of men and women. This cannot be denied. Remembering what God has done is one of the primary cures for doubt and fear.

Think about your own life and its defining moments. God would remind you:

...you were blind and lame. I opened your spiritual eyes and you walked with Me.

...I cleansed you from your sin, redeemed you, and paid the price for you.

...I led you through the darkest days of your life, and I will continue to lead you.

...I kept you together when the weight of the world came falling down.

John the Baptist was not where he expected to end up. We, too, should not expect life to be carefree. Doubt is a normal human emotion, but it should drive us closer to Christ, not away. Perseverance in the midst of a storm is essential: "You may suffer, you may bleed, you may break, but you shall go on" (Catherine Booth).

Having realistic expectations is another cure for doubt. For example, those who succeed in marriage are those who prepare for the ups and the downs. In essence, they're ready for the obstacles; they have a plan, yet remain flexible; they have expectations, but they also brace themselves for the unforeseen challenges ahead.

⇒ What is the fruit being produced by your lifestyle? What about humility; is it growing? If not, uproot pride and plant seeds of humility. God will bring stability in the midst of doubt and peace in the midst of fear.

DAY THIRTY

ARE YOU ON THE VERGE OF WRECKING YOUR LIFE?

In Russell Moore's compelling book, *Tempted & Tried*, a chapter titled, "Why You're on the Verge of Wrecking Your Life," caught my attention. Moore quotes a scientist who studied the behavior of cattle. Apparently, scientists devised a new technology that revolutionized death in the large slaughterhouses: "The cows aren't prodded off the truck but are led, in silence, onto a ramp. They go through a 'squeeze chute', a gentle pressure device that mimics a mother's nuzzling touch. The cattle continue down the ramp onto a smoothly curving path. There are no sudden turns."

He continues, "The cows experience the sensation of going home, the same kind of way they've traveled so many times before. As they mosey along the path, they don't even notice when their hooves are no longer touching the ground. A conveyor belt slowly lifts them gently upward, and then, in the twinkling of an eye, a blunt instrument levels a surgical strike right between their eyes. They're transitioned from livestock to meat, and they're never aware enough to be alarmed by any of it."

This is difficult to read but necessary. It is a vivid visual for spiritual warfare. Succumbing to temptation is often gradual, easy, and effortless until the enemy levels a surgical strike right to the heart. As I said before, we're often too smart to take deliberate plunges, but we're easily enticed to take one step at a time, one compromise at a time, one bad choice at a time until we're at the bottom keenly aware of our gradual, but deep descent.

When we obey God, He strengthens us. When we humble ourselves, His grace is manifested more abundantly, "Just as water ever seeks and fills the lowest place, so the moment God finds you abased and empty, His glory and power flow in" (Andrew Murray). Disobedience leads to desperation and despair.

Too many are choosing therapy over obedience, counseling over conduct, and talking over doing. An African pastor was asked, "Why is there so much counseling in the American church but not in the African church?" He responded, "In America you counsel; in Africa we repent." Well said.

Counseling by those who are knowledgeable and skilled in the Word is invaluable and desperately needed, but all the counseling in the world will not work if the heart is not right. God heals us primarily through our obedience to His Word and our repentance through a broken heart: "He sent His Word and healed them, and delivered them from their destructions" (Psalm 107:20). Disobedience never leads to victory. We must stop fighting this fact.

⇒ If you're on the precipice of wrecking your life, humble yourself and ask for help and direction. Our sins will find us out if we remain quiet (Numbers 32:23). Remember the key points I made in an earlier *reflection*: You'll be amazed at what God can do with humility, brokenness, and repentance. You may not be able to change your circumstances immediately, but God can get you back on the right track.

DAY THIRTY-ONE

THERE IS ANOTHER IN THE FIRE WITH YOU

In a sermon preached at a local stadium that you can find in the footnote, I said that there is no hindrance too great, no battle too hard, and no power too strong to overpower God.[1] Nothing can thwart His plans. We can take great comfort in that, but what do you do when you're going through the fire—through the trial?

We can learn a lot from the historical account of King Nebuchadnezzar in Daniel 3, who made an image of gold and told the people to bow down to it. Whoever disobeyed was cast into the midst of a fiery furnace. Shadrach, Meshach, and Abed-Nego were accused of insurrection when they refused to follow the king's orders.

The first lesson here is that we must prepare for accusations. An accusation is a charge that you did something illegal or wrong. But the key question is always "What does God's Word say?" because *legal* is not always *lawful*. In other words, something can be legal according to the laws of a particular nation but not lawful according to God's Word.

As a result of Shadrach, Meshach, and Abed-Nego's disobedience, Nebuchadnezzar became furious and gave the command to throw them into the fire. A second lesson from this narrative is that rage is often a demonic response when some don't get their way. No one can successfully debate against the truth, so those who oppose you will get upset and throw a temper tantrum.

When the three young men decided to rebel, they backed it with a powerful declaration: "Our God whom we serve is able to deliver us from the burning fiery furnace, and He will deliver *us* from your hand, O king." But they didn't stop there; they had true faith by adding that even if God didn't deliver them they would not obey the king (v. 17). We must have the same mindset: *God can deliver me, but even if He doesn't I will not bow to evil agendas. My following God is not contingent on what's happening to me; it's based on who He is.* Sometimes God removes you from the fire, and sometimes He walks through it with you—even to death. Trust God regardless of the outcome.

Another key lesson: The heat is often turned up to break you down. However, heat can be good if it removes impurities. When we pray, "Lord, help me develop patience and trust" (or whatever the struggle may be), often the heat is turned up so that a greater degree of brokenness occurs. Humble yourself, trust God, and move forward.

As these Hebrews surrendered to the will of God and trusted Him, God delivered them. Don't miss this. I'm still standing—as are many of you—because there is another in the fire! People will ask, "How are you still standing in the midst of divorce, in the midst of unemployment, in the midst of financial collapse, health issues, or persecution?" and we can answer, "Because there is another in the fire with me—the Son of God." But keep in mind that the enemy of our souls will taunt us just like the king taunted the Hebrews: "And who is the god who will deliver you from my hands?" (v. 15). When this happens, first remind yourself of God's promise in Isaiah 43:2, "When you pass through the waters, I will be with you," and then pray, "My heart will not fear what God has defeated."

⇒ Again, we must get to the point where we say, like Daniel's friends, "My God will deliver me, but even if He doesn't, I will not bow to the world's system or succumb to fear and false narratives." And then turn to Paul's reminder: "I have been crucified with Christ. It is no longer I who live, but Christ lives in me" (Galatians 2:20). For added encouragement, read the full-length article in the footnote.[2]

DAY THIRTY-TWO

SEVEN TIPS FOR TURBULENT TIMES

During difficult seasons we often ask, "Where is God?" The irony is that it often takes stormy seasons to turn us back toward safety. Fear can bring out the worst in us and harm our families. It's not that you or I will never fear but it's what we do with the fear that matters. We have a refuge during the storm if we will simply run to Him. I don't want to downplay challenges, but I also don't want to *amplify* fear.

How people respond to a crisis clearly reveals who or what they trust in. If you're fearful, angry, and anxious, take an inventory: Have you humbled yourself, repented of your sin, and asked God to save you? Are you trusting in God or in religion? In Christ or in your good works? There is no peace until you are right with God, which leads me to the first and most important point:

1. **Embrace God's wake-up call.** Psalm 119:67 reminds us of an essential truth: "Before I was afflicted I went astray, but now I keep Your word." Affliction via difficulties, challenges, and obstacles can lead us back to God. For example, in one fell swoop

COVID-19 dethroned all of our idols, and affliction brought many prodigal sons and daughters home.

2. **Difficulties can shape character or ruin it:** When affliction came to the writer of Psalm 119, he responded: "Teach me good judgment and knowledge" (v. 66). He was open and teachable. He knew that "many are the afflictions of the righteous" but that God would deliver (Psalm 34:19).

3. **Minimize media and maximize the moment.** For me, key verses in Psalm 119 have always been, "Turn away my eyes from looking at worthless things," and "Direct my steps by Your Word" (vv. 37, 133). Time spent in God's Word and in prayer changes your heart, realigning it with His. Maximize the moment and allow your relationship with God to grow and flourish. When you meditate on God's numerous promises, you are built up and encouraged rather than weakened and deflated. This leads me to point four.

4. **Fuel hope, not fear**. Psalm 119 says: "Remember the word to Your servant, upon which You have caused me to hope. This is my comfort in my affliction, for Your word has given me life" (vv. 49-50). Fear and chaos need a host (you or me), and they need fuel. You choose what you're feeding and fueling yourself with (see point three). Take this point seriously—this is where either success or failure prevails.

5. **We must persevere in prayer:** Psalm 119:147 says, "I rise before the dawning of the morning and cry for help." Persevere means to persist despite contrary influences, opposition, or discouragement. In other words, keep fighting even when the battle is getting discouraging. This is not the time to give in but to fight and to persevere. In return, you build faith, spiritual strength, and trust.

6. **Keep building; keep trusting.** The psalmist said, "My soul faints for Your salvation, but I hope in Your word" (119:81). In other words, as it becomes more and more difficult, we must keep trusting and persevering. Your family, marriage, and faith will be tested, but God is an ever-present help in times of trouble (Psalm 46:1).

7. **Cry out to God.** In the book of Joel, great swarms of locusts had devoured the land, and the people's provisions had dried up and withered away (1:4-12). They were desperate and despondent as their hope vanished. But God didn't give up on them. He told Joel to tell the people to consecrate a fast—this showed the magnitude of their sin and the need for desperation—and to come together to a sacred assembly, which represented the incredible power of unity. Then finally, they were to go into God's house and cry out to Him (1:13-14; 2:12-17). The crying out via repentance became their all-consuming priority, and it needs to be ours as well.

⇒ In what ways can you apply all seven tips to your life? I would also encourage you to read the full article where this excerpt came from in the footnote. The original title was *Overcoming Fear & Conquering Chaos: 10 Tips for Turbulent Times*.[1] Start with prayer, then make the changes that God is convicting you about.

DAY THIRTY-THREE

IS YOUR BLESSING WAITING ON YOU?

"There is a sense in which God's promises are unconditional, in that our disobedience will not thwart God's intention to be gracious, but there is also a sense in which those promises will be released only through the obedience of God's people" (Paul Carter).

The Bible is clear that God blesses His people, but it's also clear that some blessings have conditions: "If you do this, I will do that." Sadly, motivational preachers, teachers, and pastors only focus on the blessings of God without showing the other side of the coin. They say, "I have to keep my members happy and encouraged." Yes, we should encourage, but we also must convict and confront if we are to be faithful ministers of the gospel.

Many come to church praising God but not prevailing with Him, worshiping but not walking in His promises, and praying but not seeing His power because of unrepentant sin: "Your iniquities have separated you from your God; your sins have hidden his face from you, so that he will not hear" (Isaiah 59:2). As it's been said, "It is possible to have a saved soul but a lost life."

When we speak of the attributes of God, we must remember that no one attribute is greater than another and no single truth of Scripture is truer than another. To genuinely help people, we must avoid the temptation to cherry-pick. For example, Jeremiah 5:25 is powerful and heart-wrenching, and shouldn't be avoided: "Your iniquities have turned these *things* away, and your sins have withheld good from you."

He goes on to say in verses 30 and 31: "An astonishing and horrible thing has been committed in the land: The prophets prophesy falsely, and the priests rule by their *own* power; and My people love to have it so. But what will you do in the end?" False teachers are often a judgment on false converts and on those who love to have their ears tickled but not their hearts changed.[1]

When people follow their own plans, they walk backward, not forward. Disobeying God is a recurring theme from Genesis to Revelation and from the church in Acts to the church today. We must be relentless in our pursuit of God, ruthless in rooting out and dealing with our sin, and quick to repent and seek the restoration of our fellowship with God when we fail.

God's Word is clear: Blessings are hindered because of a sinful lifestyle. Whether it's wine tasting at Bible studies, promoting craft beers at men's conferences, or an array of other missteps, the Las Vegas Christian is only concerned with pleasure and ease. They "sit down to eat and drink, and rise up to play." *Sin fascinates before it assassinates!* But be encouraged—there is a way out, a way back to God—and that way out is *repentance*.

To hit disobedience right between the eyes, we must "go back to the old paths"—the old paths of holiness and deep hunger for righteousness. This forward motion leads to the filling of the Spirit. You can't be filled with disobedience and the Spirit at the same time. But even when we are obeying and being blessed, there is always a fight.

A.W. Pink, in *Gleanings from Joshua,* said: "It would indeed be strange if we apprehended how that on the one hand Canaan was a free gift unto Israel, which they entered by grace alone; and on the other, that they had to fight for every inch of it!" Blessings come with a cost; there is often a price to pay.

⇒ Are there any areas in your life where you need to "go back to the old paths"? If you agree with this statement, what changes are you willing to make today: *You can't be filled with disobedience and the Spirit at the same time.*

DAY THIRTY-FOUR

FIVE WAYS TO PREVAIL IN PRAYER

The desperate email read, *"My prayers are not being answered. I am so discouraged. Can you help?"* Although we don't fully understand God's sovereignty and its relationship to prayer, we can gain much wisdom and many truths from Scripture. Below are seven ways to prevail in prayer, taken from the sermon titled, "Travail Before You Prevail.

1. Change your spiritual diet. Psalm 5 opens with these powerful words: "Give ear to my words, O Lord, Consider my meditation" (v. 1). *Meditation* means to reflect on, to study, and to practice. Prevailing prayer begins here. What you "reflect on" creates a hunger for more. Are you meditating on the things of the world—traumatized by the news and addicted to social media—or are you meditating throughout the day on God's truth? Are you also "practicing" what the Bible says about being a doer and not just a hearer of the Word (cf. James 1:22)? What you meditate on and how you live deeply affects your prayer life.

2. Often, you must travail before you prevail. Psalm 5:2 says, "Give heed to the voice of my cry, my King and my God, for to You I will pray." In short, David is saying, "Oh God, please listen!" As in pregnancy, there is travail before the blessing. The same holds true in prayer: We must persevere, because some strongholds and many blessings are only brought about through gut-wrenching, soul-searching prayer. When we travail in prayer, God hears the cries of His children. Don't you, as a parent, run outside when you hear your children crying for help? Travail tells God that this is important; that you will do whatever it takes to see the prodigal come home, the marriage restored, or the healing takes place. No, I don't believe that God heals everyone, but I do believe that travailing prayer goes a lot further than lifeless prayer. "It is only when the whole heart is gripped with the passion of prayer that the life-giving fire descends, for none but the earnest man gets access to the ear of God" (E. M. Bounds).[1]

3. Prayer must be a priority. Verse 3 adds, "My voice You shall hear in the morning, O Lord; in the morning I will direct *it* to You, and I will look up." D. Martyn Lloyd-Jones would often tell aspiring preachers, "Safeguard your mornings!" That truth not only pertains to the pulpit but also to the pew. Whatever hurts our praying must be removed. "The men who have done the most for God in this world have been early on their knees. He who fritters away the early morning, its opportunity and freshness, in other pursuits than seeking God will make poor headway seeking Him the rest of the day" (E. M. Bounds).

Do you wake up and immediately look at your phone or social media? Are you scrambling to get out the door? My advice is to get to bed earlier and read things at night that build you up spiritually, not pull you down.

4. Remind yourself often who God is. Verses 4 and 5 appear to shift gears: "For You are not a God who takes pleasure in wickedness, nor shall evil dwell with You. The boastful shall not stand in Your sight; You hate all workers of iniquity." Reminding ourselves who God is helps us focus on His sovereignty, and it also allows us to realign our hearts by repenting of besetting sin. Ongoing and unconfessed sin kills prayer in the same way that water quenches fire.

5. Remind yourself often how good God is. Verses 6 and 7 proclaim, "You shall destroy those who speak falsehood; the Lord abhors the bloodthirsty and deceitful man. But as for me, I will come into Your house in the multitude of Your mercy; in fear of You I will worship toward Your holy temple." As the hymn "Amazing Grace" says, "It is grace that has brought me here thus far, and grace will lead me home." Meditating on the goodness of God leads to a very thankful heart, and a thankful heart is a praying heart. No one can pray well when they are bitter and resentful. Our attitudes affect our prayers more than we realize.

Many years ago, a very old man who experienced a massive revival when he was younger was asked why the revival ended. His eyes were filled with fire when he cried out, "When you lay hold of God, never, never, never, never let go!"

⇒ The same call goes out today. When God brings change, prayer has been the catalyst. The depth of God's blessings is in direct proportion to the depth of our prayer life. Prayer matters; it fuels the flames of revival. Begin to schedule prayer into your day. You won't be disappointed.

DAY THIRTY-FIVE

TRAITS OF FALSE PROPHETS
PART 1

"Then many false prophets will rise up and deceive many. And because lawlessness will abound, the love of many will grow cold" (Matthew 24:11-12).

Theologians debate the historical context of this verse, but one thing we do know is that it definitely applies today. Many people want to know about end-times signs, but first, we need to discern end-times voices—voices of truth versus those of falsehood.

Because this is such an important topic, especially today, I have included the full-length article and divided it into two parts. I also included the link for the full article in the footnote.[1]

In these dire times, many of us can relate to the prophet Jeremiah's words: "My heart within me is broken because of the [false] prophets; all my bones shake . . .because of the Lord, and because of His holy words" (Jeremiah 23:9). The lies of Israel's leaders led to Jeremiah's broken heart as well as a loss of balance and stability. God declared, "'For both prophet and priest are profane; yes, in My house I have found their wickedness,' says the Lord"

(23:11). The land, not unlike ours today, was full of unrepentant sin and fake voices, and the people were paying the price—the pleasant places were dried up.

In short, a false prophet is one who proclaims, "This is what God says," when it's not what God is saying at all. False prophets also embrace ungodly movements because they are filled with the world rather than God's Spirit. Leaders who are not filled with God's Spirit may exhibit some of the same characteristics as false prophets, which I've outlined below. However, in these cases, they lack holy fire but aren't necessarily false leaders.

A false prophet is unconverted, whereas those who are wishy-washy may simply be quenching and grieving the Spirit by their choices. Be careful in labeling people too quickly. The false prophet will draw clear lines in the sand; on the other hand, those who are struggling may just need biblical direction. If we don't cling to the cross and seek God daily, we could easily become lukewarm and not boldly stand for Him. We all must be vigilant.[2]

Although the main focus here is on those who say they believe in Jesus, there are also false prophets in cults who downright reject the deity of Christ. The apostle Peter warned, "But there were also false prophets among the people, even as there will be false teachers among you, who will secretly bring in destructive heresies, even denying the Lord who bought them, and bring on themselves swift destruction" (2 Peter 2:1). False prophets will *say* they believe in Jesus, but they've never repented of their sin and embraced him as Lord and Savior. This point is critical—just because someone says something does not mean they believe it. Always look at the fruit.

With that said, here are seven surefire signs of a false prophet based on Jeremiah 23:

1. False prophets scatter God's flock rather than unite it. "'Woe to the shepherds who destroy and scatter the sheep of My pasture!' says the Lord" (v. 1). As just one example of many, during the COVID-19 pandemonium, I saw a pastor (who I believe to be a false teacher) mock another church that had stepped out in faith to host a meeting. Sadly, some people from that church did come down with the virus. But instead of praying for the church and protecting them by not spreading gossip, the mocking pastor had the audacity to ridicule them on social media even further, thus creating division instead of unity.

False prophets also divide the body of Christ by embracing liberal theology and supporting such things as gay marriage. Spirit-filled believers are left baffled and confused because false teachers keep promoting sin rather than looking to what God says. Granted, some Christians do not fully understand what the Bible says about certain topics and may therefore appear vague on their stance. These people are not necessarily false prophets; they are biblically illiterate.

2. False prophets do not care for the spiritual needs of others. They appear loving to the world, but mature Christians can spot their hypocrisy a mile away. They march with ungodly movements but say nothing about the murdering of children in the womb. They are arrogant and boldly shake their fists at God in the name of *tolerance*. In 2 Timothy, Paul warns about people who are rebellious yet have a *form* of godliness. The world loves these false prophets because their messages do not bring conviction.

It's a given that most of us struggle with selfishness, but the rebuke from God is focused on how they lead: "'You have scattered My flock, driven them away, and not attended to them. Behold, I will attend to you for the evil of your doings,' says the

Lord" (v. 2). To not attend to their flocks is to not care for their spiritual needs.

⇒ People are dying spiritually, and false leaders counsel them to keep sinning. *Instead of offering the cure, they encourage the disease.* How can you be different and avoid wrong counsel? Hint—stay in God's Word. This leads right to the next *reflection*.

DAY THIRTY-SIX

TRAITS OF FALSE PROPHETS
PART 2

Picking up where we left off in Part One . . .

3. False leaders encourage people to indulge the flesh rather than fight it. *They are more afraid of holiness than sinfulness.* Jeremiah's words are dead on here: "They also strengthen the hands of evildoers, so that no one turns back from his wickedness" (Jeremiah 23:14). They encourage sin and avoid words like *repentance*. They won't talk about judgment because it convicts their unconverted soul. The very thing they need is the very thing they are running from—repentance. They promote freedom, but they are "slaves to depravity" (2 Peter 2:19).

There is a huge difference between a Christian who says, "I'm not really clear on this issue, but I'm searching God's Word for answers," and a leader who says that God is fine with sin. False prophets often align with Hollywood more than with the Holy Spirit. They talk about peace but never repentance: "To everyone who walks according to the dictates of his own heart, they say,

'No evil shall come upon you'" (Jeremiah 23:17). Granted, it's biblical to encourage and help people. We are to encourage them *in the midst of* their sin, but we should never *encourage sin*.

4. False prophets avoid the difficult truths in the Bible. To truly help people, we must preach the difficult truths as well as the joyful ones, preach the cross and the new life, preach hell and heaven, preach damnation and salvation, preach sin and grace, preach wrath and love, preach judgment and mercy, preach obedience and forgiveness, preach that God is love but not forget that God is just. It is the love of God that compels us to share all His truth. But false teachers avoid unpleasant doctrines because they would rather tickle the ears of their hearers rather than challenge their hearts. *Christians should not be an echo chamber for the world but a powerful voice proclaiming God's Word with a spirit of humility.*

5. False prophets use the phrase "don't judge" out of context. To them, "judge not" apparently means "don't offend." When asked why they don't ever talk about sin, their reasons go something like this: "It's not my job to judge, just to love." Yes, we need to love people and avoid a judgmental attitude, but this isn't the issue here. Leonard Ravenhill was famous for saying that we must "weep before we whip." True, biblical love speaks the truth, especially regarding moral issues that destroy lives and dishonor God. We are to judge, to "call into question" behaviors, choices, and lifestyles that lead people in a dangerous direction. In 1 Corinthians 2:15, the apostle Paul said that those who are spiritual should judge and discern all things. Jesus's famous words "judge not" were meant to condemn a pride-filled judgmental heart, not to have us remain silent on sin. Simply read Matthew 7 in its full context.

6. False prophets question the inerrancy and reliability of Scripture. As a result, they often say, "I think," rather than "I know" when it comes to biblical truth. This is where the trouble starts. When we minimize the authority of God's Word and maximize our opinion, we will always lead others astray. False teachers have no solid foundation for their lives or for their theology. But "if they had stood in My counsel, and had caused My people to hear My words, then they would have turned them from their evil way and from the evil of their doings" (Jeremiah 23:22). God is crystal clear here that only the undiluted preaching of His Word leads to radically changed lives. Ironically, even though they question God's Word, they don't like to be questioned. Truth invites scrutiny, but error runs from it.

7. False prophets lack boldness and have no urgency in their preaching. When God truly calls a person and fills them with His Spirit, boldness always follows. They speak with authority and urgency. They are more concerned about God's opinion than popular opinion. This is what the Lord says: "Stand in the courtyard of the LORD's house and . . .tell them everything I command you; do not omit a word" (Jeremiah 26:2).

Yes, love and grace have conquered many hard hearts, but God also uses bold preaching: "'Is not My word like a fire?' says the Lord, 'And like a hammer that breaks the rock in pieces?'" (Jeremiah 23:29). But false teachers "speak great swelling *words* of emptiness" and "they allure through the lusts of the flesh" (2 Peter 2:18). *Their words are not a burning fire but empty pleasantries.*

True prophetic voices are often too radical for most people because they threaten their comfort zone and dismantle lukewarm Christianity. But isn't that the whole point? "When we become so tolerant that we lead people into mental fog and spiritual darkness, we are not acting like Christians—we are acting like cowards" (A.W. Tozer).

⇒ The most important question one can face is, "Do you truly know God?" We cannot minimize the destruction, danger, and damage of sin. Jesus didn't die on the cross for a minor violation. He died because the wrath of God was abiding on every human who ever lived. If you're a false teacher, or if you've drifted from God, please change that today, and embrace the wonderful gift of assurance obtained through repentance and confession of sin. "If the Son makes you free, you shall be free indeed" (John 8:36). God's grace will flood your soul as He renews and rebuilds your life.

DAY THIRTY-SEVEN

DEALING WITH DEPRESSION AND MENTAL ILLNESS

Many know all too well the debilitating effects of mental illness. We do a great disservice when we tell those struggling to "just get over it and think positive thoughts" or "read your Bible more." Although positive thinking (the right kind) is biblical, and it's crucial to meditate on God's Word, one cannot simply turn depression, anxiety, and hopelessness on and off like a light switch. But it's also important to recognize that there are factors that contribute to mental anguish.

After many years of praying with, talking to, and counseling thousands of people, I've found five factors that stand out that may cause mental pain.[1] I also recommend reading the full article in the footnote where this excerpt first appeared.[2]

1. Chemical imbalances and other physical factors can cause mental illness. Medication has a place, such as when neurotransmitters and hormone levels need correction. In the same way that diabetes needs to be treated with insulin, some struggling with emotional pain may need medication such as serotonin reuptake inhibitors, but medication doesn't always fix the problem.

2. The consequences of besetting sin can cause mental pain. In Psalm 32:3 (NASB), David said, "When I kept silent about my sin, my body wasted away through my groaning all day long." Living life outside of God's will or being unrepentant in relation to besetting sin can lead to mental anguish, depression, and anxiety. Life can be very complex, and sometimes there are no easy or instant solutions to the problems we experience, but it's always wise to examine our problems in the light of God's Word. Repentance can bring peace with God and healing to our spirit.

3. A toxic diet can affect mental health. No surprise here . . . what's eating you may have to do with what you're eating. Most people know that poor food choices affect *physical* health, but they fail to see the connection with *mental* health. Over the years I've noticed that those suffering from depression rarely eat healthy (of course there are exceptions). Usually, their diet consists of things such as potato chips and soft drinks, rather than large colorful salads. In many cases, there is definitely a connection. How many are suffering simply because of poor food choices?[3]

4. A demonic attack can affect mental health. We can't rule out the possibility of a spiritual attack. Throughout the New Testament, demonic activity caused mental anguish. If a person takes high-powered drugs, they may only increase the problem and could open the door to further demonic activity. *Pharmakeía* (from where we get our word *pharmacy*) means to administer drugs. In the Bible, it was often tied to the practice of magic and sorcery. Medication for depression can sometimes cause suicidal thoughts. It's an area we need to be careful in.

Have you opened any obvious doors such as palm reading, tarot cards, alcohol, drugs, or Ouija boards? Is there a family history of occult practices? If so, have those who are strong in the faith pray for you regularly. *Sometimes strongholds have to be pulled down one brick at a time.*

5. An unhealthy spiritual diet negatively affects mental health. I know that I've really been driving this home, but what are you feeding your mind? Are you fueling fear and paranoia by spending too much time listening to the media? Are you watching horror movies—especially paranormal and excessively violent ones—and other forms of ungodly entertainment? What kind of music do you listen to—uplifting and encouraging or worldly and sensual? Take time and read Philippians 4 to see what the apostle Paul has to say about our mental diet. What you put into your mind plays a huge role in your mental health.

⇒ If you find yourself trapped in addiction, misery, and depression, there is hope. God continually calls us back to Him. If you return with all your heart, He will return to you. That's a gift of the greatest value . . . a promise that will never fail. He is our only Hope. But if you've done that and have a vibrant relationship with God, yet still struggle, keep pressing on. Bouts of depression are common to most of us as a by-product of this fallen world, but the reward at the end of the race will far exceed the disappointments of this world. Don't give up. Look up!

DAY THIRTY-EIGHT

MICROWAVE CHRISTIANITY ISN'T HEALTHY

As we all know, America is in a spiritual decline with no recovery in sight. Many churches have a form of "microwave" Christianity: service times last just over an hour, prayer is glanced over, and worship is designed to entertain the masses. Many pastors avoid offending their audience and seek to motivate rather than convict. If we truly want to see revival, the face of the present-day church needs to change.

Some pastors say, "People are bored, so our services need to be more appealing." Church services are boring because the power of God has vanished from many congregations. There is a lack of desire to pursue God in both the pulpit and the pew. Like Samson, they don't realize that the Spirit of the Lord has departed (Judges 16:20). But there is hope. We can once again position ourselves to seek God: "You will seek Me and find Me when you seek Me with all your heart" (Jeremiah 29:13).

In this context, to seek means to "find what is missing." The Hebrew word for *seek*, *baqash*, has a very strong meaning.

Imagine losing your child in a crowded mall. Your entire heart would be engaged. How would you spend your time? Where would your energy be concentrated? Now parallel this with seeking God. Pastors and Christian leaders, we must again seek God as if our nation and the future of our children depend on it—because it does. Where is the weeping? Where are the early morning prayer meetings? Where is the fasting?

Remember when the church sought God in an upper room for days until fire fell? Remember when we were not in a hurry, and extended worship services drove us to our knees? Remember when seeking God through prayer drove the church? Methods, marketing programs, and surveys now lead the way. Remember when prayer and seeking God were assets, not liabilities, to church growth? Remember when people were excited about seeking God rather than busy making excuses as to why they can't attend church?

We need powerful times of prayer, devotion, and worship. *"Without the heartbeat of prayer, the body of Christ will resemble a corpse. The church is dying on her feet because she is not living on her knees"* (Al Whittinghill). Prayerlessness in the pulpit leads to apostasy and dead sermons. Prayerlessness in the pew leads to shattered lives and depression. Prayerlessness in men leads to the breakdown of the family. Prayerlessness in Washington leads to the breakdown of society.

God is not too busy, He's not on vacation, and He's not sleeping. He is an ever-present help in time of need. You can call out to Him in the deep of the night or in the midst of the storm. He hears the prayers of His children, but we must once again cultivate a life of seeking Him through prayer, brokenness, obedience, and humility.

A word of caution though: we can humble ourselves, pray, and seek His face, but all this will fall on deaf ears unless we turn from our wicked ways: "Surely the arm of the Lord is not too short to save, nor His ear too dull to hear. But your iniquities have separated you from your God; your sins have hidden His face from you, so that He will not hear" (Isaiah 59:1–2).

We must turn from our rebellion, including idols that have diverted our passion for Christ. He came that we might be free from the bondage of sin, not continue in it. We must understand that we cannot flaunt sin in the face of God without consequence.

Social media is filled with jealousy and envy, and a competitive spirit permeates many aspects of our lives. Self-indulgence is rampant in the church. Sexual sin has become an epidemic. Many churches add gimmicks and dumb down the gospel in an attempt to reach the culture, but the pulpit is to be sacred, not secular. And we wonder why the American church has drifted off course, why we're not experiencing powerful moves of God? *Most churches resemble a social gathering rather than a powerful worship service.*

The truth is that we have "perverted the words of the living God" (Jeremiah 23:36) by not warning and challenging people to turn from their sin. Pastors, as the church falls deeper into self-reliance and further from reliance on God, its need for bold leadership has never been greater. Life-changing sermons must come from a man whose life has been changed by God. Change will only occur in America when there is a strong conviction of sin and sincere repentance—may God grant us the wisdom and strength to proclaim these truths.

. . .

⇒ Are you confusing God's patience with His approval? You must take seriously His call to return. Do that now by acknowledging your drift from God and your willingness to change. Ask Him to strengthen and empower you.

DAY THIRTY-NINE

SURVIVING THE ANOINTING

The word *anointing* has been used and abused by charlatans and schemers, but the word is thoroughly biblical. An anointing happens when God fills a person with His Spirit for the purpose of using him or her in a mighty way. In the time of Samson, Israel was in bondage, and God anointed Samson as a judge and a deliverer. God's anointing is absolutely necessary for accomplishing His will. Make no mistake, our families and our nation need more men and women anointed by God.[1]

Here are a few lessons from Samson's life that can help along the way. The full article is in the footnote.[2]

Survive the anointing by knowing Who to run to when pressured. Judges 16:16 says that Delilah "pestered him daily with her words and pressed him, so that his soul was vexed to death." When Samson was beaten down and worn out, "he told her all his heart, and said to her, 'No razor has ever come upon my head, for I have been a Nazirite to God from my mother's womb. If I am shaven, then my strength will leave me, and I shall become weak, and be like any other man'" (v. 17). *His power was not in his hair, but in his consecration to the Lord.* The same is true for us—spiritual power is found in obedience and consecration.

Survive the anointing by guarding your heart. In verses 18–19 we read, "When Delilah saw that he had told her all his heart, she sent and called for the lords of the Philistines, saying, 'Come up once more, for he has told me all his heart.'" Then she lulled him to sleep and called for a man to shave his hair. Samson should have fled her presence once he noticed her deception in prior encounters. Sin lulls us to sleep via compromise and complacency. As I said before, *Sin fascinates, then assassinates.* You can't defeat your demons if you're still enjoying their company!

Survive the anointing by staying humble. You'd be amazed at what God does with humility and equally amazed at how much pride blocks His blessings. The Apostle Peter warns us that *"God resists the proud, but gives grace to the humble"* (1 Peter 5:5). The Bible illustrates this principle in the story of Samson and Delilah. It shows us Samson's mindset when he woke up: "And she said, 'The Philistines are upon you, Samson!' So he awoke from his sleep, and said, 'I will go out as before, at other times, and shake myself free!'" (Judges 16:20). He must have thought, "I can handle this; I've got this. I'm Samson, the mighty man of God." Samson was trusting in his own strength, but "he did not know that the Lord had departed from him" (v. 20).

Survive the anointing by staying focused on the goal while waiting on God. In verse 21, we read that the Philistines took him and put out his eyes. They bound him, and he became a grinder in the prison. Spiritual eyesight keeps us focused in the right direction, which is why clouding our vision is one of the enemy's favorite tactics: "You will grope at noon, as the blind man gropes in darkness, and you will not prosper in your ways" (Deut. 28:29). But don't give up—an incredible transformation appears in the next verse: "However, the hair of his head began to grow again." As Samson no doubt repented and prayed and trusted again in God, his strength came back. The same holds true for us. Wait on God, pray, and seek His face. Waiting time is not wasted time.[3]

Survive the anointing by remembering who you are, even when others taunt you. Samson was brought into a large arena to be taunted by the Philistines. They laughed and jeered at his apparent defeat. Tauntings come during seasons of victory and defeat, during mountaintop experiences and low valleys, when you're doing God's will and when you've fallen. Expect them, and prepare for them accordingly by remembering who will see you through: *"Through many dangers, toils, and snares I have already come; 'tis grace hath brought me safe thus far, and grace will lead me home."* Enemies of God will always taunt us, but that's all they can do. God always gets the last word.

7. Survive the anointing by knowing where to put your hands. Samson took hold of the two pillars that supported the temple, and he braced himself against them. Then Samson cried out "Let me die with the Philistines!" And he pushed with all his might, and the temple fell on the people who were in it. Like Samson, you too can recapture your focus, renew your strength, and finish your race.

. . .

⇒ If you're facing a time of despair, put your feet on the neck of the enemy, and pull down the pillars of bondage and sin through heart-wrenching prayer and deep repentance: "Oh God, remember me. Strengthen me to fight again!"[4]

DAY FORTY

WHY REVIVAL IS AMERICA'S ONLY HOPE!

Since a spiritual awakening is often conceived in prayer and birthed in fasting, I couldn't think of a better way to end this book than with this final reflection of the full-length article (the longest of the forty daily reflections). The link to share it on social media is in the footnote for ebook users.[1]

The results are in: America's stage four cancer has metastasized to the family and the church as well as to the government and the schools. We are more depraved than ever before. Animals are guarded but innocent children are slaughtered. Porn is protected and sex trafficking is on the rise. Cardi B's lyrics get a pass but Scriptures are banned on social media.

Words cannot express this outright lunacy. Like the bungee jumper who plunged to her death because she thought she heard "now jump," when, in reality, her instructor said, "No jump!" America thinks that she is hearing from God, but she is not. We are drowning in a cesspool of moral filth: "The wicked freely parade and prance about while evil is praised throughout the land" (Psalm 12:8).

Recently, a father was arrested for referring to his biological 14-year-old daughter as "she" after she transitioned to a male gender.[2] "But that's in Canada," you say. Trust me, we are not far behind. Most on the liberal left would have no problem imprisoning anyone who disagreed with them, and that's exactly where the Equality Act is going—unless you accept, rejoice in, and validate sin they are coming after you. Revival is our only hope.

We see throughout the Bible that there is only one remedy—one solution—one cure to reverse the judgment of God: *Revival*. During times of crisis, the cure for judgment was to return back to God: "Consecrate a fast, call a sacred assembly; gather the elders and all the inhabitants of the land into the house of the Lord your God, and cry out to the Lord" (Joel 1:14).

Revival changes a nation from the inside out. Benjamin Franklin, commenting on George Whitefield's preaching, said this about the revival sweeping the land, "It was wonderful to see the change soon made in the manners of our inhabitants. From being thoughtless or indifferent about religion, it seemed as if all the world were growing religious." Revival must begin in the pulpits as well as the pews.

Revival is not adding more church services to the calendar. Revival is not having a guest speaker host an event. And revival most certainly is not acting weird and loud. Revival is a sovereign act of God: "Wilt thou not revive us again: that thy people may rejoice in thee?" (Psalm 85:6).

In the same way that we cannot produce a bumper crop by making it rain, revival cannot be planned, organized, or scheduled, but you can till the soil of your heart: "I live in a high and holy place, but also with the one who is contrite and lowly in spirit, to revive the spirit of the lowly and to revive the heart of the contrite" (Isaiah 57:15).

Revival is when we till the soil through brokenness, humility, and surrender via fasting and prayer. God responds by rending the heavens with a downpour: "Oh, that you would rend the heavens and come down, that the mountains would tremble before you" (Isaiah 64:1)!

As stated earlier, the cold hard truth is that many are not willing to pay the price. Gone are the days of John Wesley, George Whitefield, and Jonathan Edwards who would fast and pray as if America's future depended upon it (because it did and still does). It's no surprise that Edwards' famous sermon, *Sinners in the Hand of an Angry God*, was preached at the tail end of his three-day fast. Today that title would be labeled offensive and many pastors would be too ashamed to preach it—too ashamed because they lack the fire of the Spirit.

Gone are the days of David Brainard who spent nights in agonizing prayer, as well as "praying" John Hyde, William Bramwell, and countless others who prayed fervently for our nation. Instead of carrying the baton and running the race, we are captivated by *American Idol*, love our porn, and over-indulge. King Stomach is clearly on the throne.

"It's too hard to fast," we say. The problem isn't fasting; it's addiction. We can't fast because we're withdrawing from our favorite addictions: coffee, sugar, alcohol, processed food, and so on. Let that sink in. And we wonder why we aren't experiencing a massive move of God in our nation. We abort revival before it's even been conceived.

When revivals spread across our landscape, Christians spent countless hours praying and fasting. They paid the price! When pastors stood at the pulpit they preached boldly about the cross, sin, judgment, and repentance. They could say, "Thus saith the Lord," because they were filled with the Holy Spirit, not Hollywood. They didn't work revival up, God brought it down because His Word was honored.

Today, most pastors want to be popular and most Christians want their ears tickled. If you doubt this, just look at the top sermons on social media today and their attire. The messages are soothing rather than convicting. As in Israel's day, the people still say, "You must not prophesy to us what is right! Speak to us pleasant things and smooth words, prophesy [deceitful] illusions [that we will enjoy]" (Isaiah 30:10 AMP).

Granted, we need to hear uplifting messages, but we have a huge problem when pastors don't want to ruffle feathers and Christians don't want to hear controversial topics. America's stage four cancer was caused by a bad diet of frivolous preaching. The cure will require a complete diet change back to whole life-giving food from the Word of God.

I don't say this in arrogance; my heart breaks for the church. This is more of a plea than a rebuke, but the truth is, "We have too many puppets in our pulpits and not enough prophets" (Leonard Ravenhill). Pastors and Christians must lead the way, but the way won't be popular and wide, it will be narrow and difficult. We must fast like it matters, pray like we mean it, and seek God as if everything depends upon it, because it does.

Nearly a decade ago, I prayed, "Lord, bring revival to the churches," but I was not ready for the response that followed. I share the response and the sermon below as often as possible to reach as many people as possible.

After I prayed, it was almost as if God was saying: "You don't want revival—it will ruin your schedule, your dignity, your image, and your reputation as a person who is 'well balanced.' Men will weep throughout the congregation. Women will wail because of the travail of their own souls. Young adults will cry like children at the magnitude of their sin. With the strength of My presence, the worship team will cease playing. Time will seem to stand still. You won't be able to preach because of the emotions flooding your own soul. You'll struggle to find words, but only find tears. Even the most dignified and reserved among you will be broken and humbled as little children. The proud and self-righteous will not be able to stand in My presence. The doubter and unbeliever will either run for fear or fall on their knees and worship Me—there can be no middle ground. The church will never be the same again."

⇒ Do you truly want revival? It will cost you. National revival begins with personal revival when we look in the mirror, repent, and turn toward God. *He is our only hope.* Watch the sermon, *The True Cost of Revival,* in the footnote.[3]

APPENDIX: MY DAILY FASTING BREAKDOWN

Below are some of my daily/weekly experiences during the first two weeks of the fast. During the first week, I recorded a day-to-day overview followed by weekly experiences. My hope is that outlining this journey will give you a glimpse into what to expect. I also recorded a video of this experience. The link is in the footnote.[1]

DAY ONE: *Not Too Bad*—I wasn't too hungry on day one; the power of the made-up mind helped. I slept over seven hours. Spiritually I felt blah.

DAY TWO: *Mr. Moody*—I was moody all day. Not only was my body detoxing, but my flesh didn't like the idea of not having food. I was hungry throughout the day. This was a key day for me: Would I give up or fight? Thankfully, I made it to the evening and fell asleep by 8:30 p.m. I had another good night's sleep. I also began to feel cold (it lasted throughout the entire fast).

DAY THREE: *Feel the Burn*—Day three wasn't too eventful, but a simple ketone test revealed that I was finally burning a moderate amount of fat as my primary fuel source. (The test strips are available at most drug stores.) If ketones don't stay high during a fast, it could be because your cells are adapting to them, thus lowering the amount of ketones in the urine.

Fasting became really challenging toward the end of the day. I almost caved in, but fortunately, I fell asleep. Staying focused on getting through the first three days helped. Spiritually speaking, the last few days were challenging.

DAY FOUR: *Pain Has a Purpose*—I began to feel pain in my lower back and right knee that lasted for days. The pain, in all likelihood, was caused by *retracing*. The body often retraces past problems in order to heal them. For example, if you had a cold some time back, you might see those same symptoms again while the body is healing.

Even though I had lost ten pounds (most of which was water and glycogen), I felt like I was filled with concrete. Even simple movements took significant energy. Keeping my eyes focused on the goals mentioned earlier kept me going. I didn't feel good on this day so I had some bone broth and a small protein shake.

DAY FIVE: *Still Spiritually Dry*—Although I was maintaining spiritual disciplines over the last few days, my prayers felt dry and my desire to read the Word was fading. Recall what I said earlier: *When you don't feel good physically (there are exceptions), you often don't feel good spiritually.*

Up to this point, the fast wasn't what I had hoped for spiritually speaking, but that's to be expected because God "is a rewarder of those who diligently seek Him" (Hebrews 11:6). The context of this verse focuses on moving forward despite how we *feel* or what we see: "Without faith it is impossible to please Him, for he who comes to God must believe that He is, and that He is a rewarder of those who diligently seek Him." With the Lord's help, I made it this far, and there was no way I was going to quit now. Perseverance and fortitude lead to motivation.

DAY SIX: *Cherishing the Change*—An incredible thing happened: I couldn't stop writing as God downloaded a powerful article into my heart. The title was, *Why Revival is America's Only Hope!* It's located on day forty of the daily reflections. For those who'd like to share the article, the link is in the footnote.[2]

Physically speaking, I finally started to feel better even though my mouth had a weird taste and I was weak and sore. Even though I had lower back and joint pain, my body was more flexible. Just for fun, I did fifty push-ups fairly easily. Ironically, just a few weeks ago, I couldn't hit fifty. It is difficult to watch strength plummet as we age. I bench-pressed 400 pounds in my early twenties but can't do much today due to my shoulder and elbow injuries.

Additionally, periodic urinalysis tests showed that I had high levels of leukocytes over the last few months. A high reading means that the white blood cell count is high so the body can fight an infection. When I checked the

levels today, I was happy that they were back down to normal. *This was very encouraging because I wasn't sure how (or where) the infection originated, but I know how it ended: Fasting.*

I still felt bland and monotone physically as well as spiritually, but I kept reminding myself of the biblical concept of *delayed* gratification.

DAY SEVEN: *Light at the End of the Tunnel*—What a morning. I only had about five hours of sleep because I was restless until

11:00 p.m., but God met me this morning in a powerful way. I couldn't stop worshiping. See the footnote for two of my favorites songs during this season.[3]

Physically speaking, ketones were still high but a urinalysis test also showed high levels of *specific gravity*. High specific gravity levels could indicate dehydration and low electrolytes, so I increased my water intake and added a liquid trace mineral supplement that seemed to work well. I also had decaf organic coffee and herbal tea with no sweetener from time to time throughout the week.

THE SECOND WEEK: Going into this second week, my morning time was incredible. I woke up around 4 a.m. with renewed excitement to spend a few hours listening to worship and reading God's Word. There were solemn times as well as times when I couldn't stop crying. Oh, if I could stay in that state all day!

I was also able to write another new article titled, *A Battle Cry for a Dead Church*.[4] Additionally, I couldn't stop listening to worship and meditating on God's Word. God kept pouring love and brokenness into my heart as I felt the weight of how far our nation and the church have drifted from Him.

I felt good every morning and woke up refreshed, but one of the most difficult challenges for me was the extra time that I had. When I wasn't eating or preparing to eat or making something to eat or driving to get something to eat, I had a few extra hours each day. Instead of lunch and dinner with family and friends, I had to stay busy doing different things. For example, I often read books, went on walks, and worked on this book. It was hard altering my lifestyle because so much of it was tied to food, but by the second week, I looked forward to these times of retreat.

MY TOP TEN HEALTH TIPS

My hope is that you continue to use this book and apply the forty day reset when you feel the need. Focusing on the ten tips below can greatly improve physical health. These tips were pulled directly from the opening chapters, and are designed to be printed, posted, and shared.

I also added a *daily checklist*. If you're not able to fulfill some of the commitments on the daily checklist, start again the next day.

1. Focus on eating God-given, living plant food as your primary fuel source rather than boxed and processed dead food. Limit even healthy meat and dairy.

2. Resist the temptation to eat frequently such as snacking throughout the day. Stop when satisfied rather than full, and consider fasting intermittently throughout the week.

3. Incorporate fasting into your yearly routine with long fasts once or twice a year, or shorter fasts quarterly. Try weekly fasts such as not eating for twenty-four hours now and then.

4. Make sure to get enough sleep as well as rest. Without stimulants and alarm clocks, we can easily sleep seven to eight hours. Before the lightbulb was invented, most people slept at least eight hours. Remember, the body heals and repairs when we sleep.

5. Avoid stimulants such as coffee and black tea. Stimulants hinder deep sleep and add stress to our lives because they keep us in a constant state of "fight or flight."

6. Take a day off each week from social media and the negative news. Instead, use the time to seek God and rest in Him.

7. When possible, avoid unnecessary medication since most are toxic to the body. For example, those taking medication for health-related illnesses such as heart disease and type 2 diabetes, should talk to their doctor about weaning off medication by changing their diet and losing weight.

8. Stay active, whether it's daily walks, parking further away, using stairs, working in the yard, exercising with your kids, or taking bike rides. It's important to keep moving. The old adage is true: "If you don't use it you will lose it."

9. Incorporate resistance and cardiovascular training into your weekly routine. Muscle and heart strength are very important to longevity.

10. Put God first in everything you do. Make your relationship with Him *daily* a priority and everything else will fall into place.

DAILY CHECKLIST

1	2	3	4	5	6	7	8	9	10
11	12	13	14	15	16	17	18	19	20
21	22	23	24	25	26	27	28	29	30
31	32	33	34	35	36	37	38	39	40

→ Did I spend time praying?

→ Did I spend time reading God's Word?

→ Did I apply God's Word? If so, how?

→ Did I spend time reading a good book?

→ Did I make amends with those I wronged?

→ Did I make sure that my heart is right before God?

- Did I get enough sleep and rest?
- Did I deal with stress correctly and avoid stimulants?
- Did I exercise using cardio and resistance training?
- Did I drink enough water?
- Did I avoid junk food and sweets?
- Did I eat enough whole plant food?

RECOMMENDED READING

Breaking the Stronghold of Food by Dr. Michael Brown is exceptional, and it's written from a Christian perspective. It doesn't focus on fasting per se but on other important elements of a healthy diet.

Fasting Can Save Your Life by Herbert M. Shelton is recognized as one of the all-time bestsellers on fasting. This book is a valuable resource even though it was written many years ago. Science has made many advances since its first publication, but the principles are timeless.

What the Bible Says about Healthy Living by Rex Russell and *The Maker's Diet* by Jordan Rubin are compelling resources for those wanting more information regarding what the Bible says about food. They grant more liberty with eating meat than what I promote.

God's Chosen Fast by Arthur Wallis is another exceptional resource that covers a lot more than what I can cover in this short book.

Fast Your Way to Health by J. Harold Smith outlines the physical and spiritual benefits of fasting. I appreciate his simple and straightforward approach.

The Power of Prayer and Fasting by Ronnie Floyd is an encouraging book for the pulpit as well as the pew. Although he is a pastor and talks about his 40-day juice fast experience, men and women from all walks of life can benefit from this resource, especially if you're hungry for revival.

A Hunger for God by John Piper is captivating and convicting.

Fasting Can Change Your Life by Jerry Falwell and Elmer Towns will strengthen your faith by providing testimonies of contemporary Christians who fasted and reaped the benefits.

Revival Now! Through Prayer and Fasting by Gordon Cove includes examples of people who fasted in the Bible and what the outcome was—encouraging, motivating, and convicting. Part one is on prayer and part two is on fasting.

The Complete Guide to Fasting: Heal Your Body Through Intermittent, Alternate-Day, and Extended Fasting by Jimmy Moore and Dr. Jason Fung is not a biblical resource, but it is a good resource to truly understand how the body works, especially if you're struggling with diabetes, cancer, or heart disease.

Although I don't agree with Dr. Fung's stance on evolution, as I've said before: Eat the meat and throw out the bones (no pun intended for my plant-based diet friends). This book is lengthy and encourages heavy meat and fat consumption as well as the use of coffee. Although I understand where he's coming from regarding the ketogenic approach, I don't fully endorse those views either.

OTHER BOOKS BY THE AUTHOR

Links for all the books are available here.

1. ***Oh God, Would You Rend the Heavens?*** The need to address revival and the vital role of the Holy Spirit is as relevant today as it has been throughout church history. Parts one and two of this booklet focus on the importance of having the right heart; whereas parts three and four focus on the errors of conservatives as well as charismatics. My hope is that all of us, including myself, humble ourselves and find the middle ground ... the common ground.
2. ***Feasting and Fasting:*** When the body rests and is allowed to heal, many call the results *miraculous*, but this is just how God created us. Fasting not only creates an environment of health and healing, but more importantly, it facilitates spiritual growth. There are also free download links available on some of the platforms.
3. ***HELP! I'm Addicted:*** We are at the crossroads: Opioid and alcohol abuse are leaving a path of destruction in their wake. Pornography is desecrating families. Obesity is skyrocketing and plaguing millions—it has even reached epidemic levels in children. Cancer and heart disease are the number one killers in America. And on and on it goes from nicotine to caffeine to food—as a society, we are out of control. But are there answers? Yes, there are, if we once again set our sites on God's truth.

4. ***If My People:*** Hopeless headlines dominate the news cycle, and it's called *psychological warfare*, and the goal is to elevate stress to the point of exhaustion and then fuel fear so that people lose hope. To win this battle (the battle of the mind), one must saturate their mind in the Word and ways of God. The new book by Pastor Shane, *If My People,* is a cry for us to turn back to God, to seek His face, and to receive the blessings He promises to those who will humble themselves.

5. ***Desperate for More of God:*** One of the greatest joys associated with pastoring is seeing others filled with the Spirit of God—"You will seek me and find me when you seek me with all your heart" (Jeremiah 29:13). This is what I'm seeking to do in this book—to fan the flames of passion toward God.

6. ***One Nation Above God:*** "What America is and has been was the result of previous generations; everything she will become depends on the rising generation. Shane fully understands this and has provided our next generation of leaders with an understanding of the principles that will keep America great. This book can help secure America's future as 'one nation under God.'" —David Barton, President and Founder, WallBuilders, Aledo, Texas.

7. ***Answers for a Confused Church:*** "Shane Idleman rings a clarion bell for the church today, calling it to its primary duty, to proclaim the truth in the power of the Holy Spirit. The church is not called to make the Gospel acceptable but to make it clear. That is preaching the truth. Shane gives a stark reminder to the Emergent Church Movement." Alex Montoya Associate Professor of Pastoral Ministries, The Master's Seminary in Sun Valley, California.

8. ***What Works for Men:*** Whether single, married or divorced, all of us have made mistakes and have probably fallen short of our hopes and expectations. God's Word provides direction and encouragement through challenges and tough decisions; thus, a large portion of *What Works for Men* draws from biblical principles and is intended to inspire and motivate.
9. ***What Works for Young Adults:*** "Sit down, buckle up, and hold on! This is one of the best resources for young adults in the publishing industry today." Tim Wildmon, American Family Association.
10. ***What Works for Singles:*** This resource will help those who are single and looking to marry in the future, as well as those who have experienced the painful realities of divorce.
11. ***What Works When "Diet's" Don't:*** Learn what works, what doesn't, and why when it comes to losing weight and keeping it off. This book approaches weight loss from a biblical perspective and offers hope and encouragement. Diets don't work, but lifestyle changes do.

NOTES

EPIGRAPH 1

1. Quote from John Piper: https://www.desiringgod.org/interviews/reckoning-with-personal-failure.

INTRODUCTION . . . START HERE

1. Beeke and Thomas, *Pastors and Their Critics*; P&R Publishing Company, New Jersey © 2020; Pg. 168.
2. More here: https://www.lifehack.org/520861/the-cold-truth-about-the-diet-industry-america.
3. Dr. Alec Burton also uses this analogy in his message, *Fasting for Health and Recovery*, and it's a great message as well: https://www.youtube.com/watch?v=wAbZY7gEZNk.
4. Gordon Cove, *Revival Now! Through Prayer & Fasting pt. 2*, published by Rare Christian Books, pg. 3.
5. The teachings are here: https://westsidechristianfellowship.org/teachings/fasting/ and the awesome menu options are here: https://freshwholeplantiful.com/. The WCF Healthy Living Accountability & Support Group here: https://www.facebook.com/groups/637762103075304.
6. My YouTube channel is here: https://www.youtube.com/channel/UCoE2tPwSq8oTSFcKp9q-Tkw.

WHAT IS A RESET?

1. Located in Gordon Cove's short pamphlet on fasting.
2. E. Stanley Jones, *A Song of Ascents* (Nashville: Abingdon, 1979), page 383.

FOCUS ON PROGRESS, NOT PERFECTION

1. More can be found here: https://www.webmd.com/mental-health/eating-disorders/what-is-orthorexia#1.
2. The message is here: https://www.youtube.com/watch?v=sWN13pKVp9s.

3. To Be Heard On High is here: https://www.youtube.com/watch?v=S5tPxR7-8LA. When the Church Had Power is here: https://www.youtube.com/watch?v=agAH5qwQcnQ. Igniting Revival–Dead Bones Come Alive is here: https://www.youtube.com/watch?v=G318qXQWyK8.

WHY FORTY AND WHY FASTING?

1. Arthur Wallis, *God's Chosen Fast*, published by CLC Publications © 1968, pg. 9.
2. Here is more about *Post-acute Withdrawal Syndrome,* including time-lines and medical information: *https://americanaddictioncenters.org/withdrawal-timelines-treatments/post-acute-withdrawal-syndrome*
3. Dr. Joel Fuhrman, *Fasting and Eating for Health,* © 1995, St. Martin's Press, pg. 177.
4. Here is a good article that may help: To Souls Who Fall Asleep - Six Ways to Stay Awake to God.
5. Herbert M Shelton, *The Science and Fine Art of Fasting*, published by the Natural Hygiene Press © 1978, pg. 363. Edward H. Dewey also wrote about treating alcoholism with fasting in the late 1800s. The title is: *Chronic Alcoholism: Its Cure, Without Money, Without Price.*
6. For more about resting in God, read this sermon transcript from Charles Spurgeon delivered January 14th, 1877: https://www.spurgeon.org/resource-library/sermons/rest-in-the-lord/#flipbook/.
7. Watch this short clip about men being watchmen: https://www.youtube.com/watch?v=wiZtiFA4_HY
8. For added encouragement, watch this short clip titled, *How to Find Rest in Turbulent Times:* https://www.youtube.com/watch?v=rHvtUNOF7O8.
9. Listen here for *Why is the Bible So Confusing?* as well as other important topics: https://idlemanunplugged.podbean.com/e/why-is-the-bible-so-confusing-what-about-all-the-inconsistencies/
10. To spark hunger for prayer, read books on prayer by E.M. Bounds, A.W. Tozer, and Leonard Ravenhill. I have found that what I read or listen to at night affects how I feel in the morning.

FASTING APPLIES PRESSURE TO THE SPIRITUAL REALM

1. Paul Washer breaks down the importance of fasting for spiritual reasons here in under three minutes: https://www.youtube.com/watch?v=mrSEtvaGnPU
2. Wallis, *God's Chosen Fast,* 53.
3. *Atomic Power with God Through Fasting and Prayer* by Franklin Hall, published in 1946 contains a much larger list. His book is not for the average person . . . it's pretty intense, and a little dated.

4. Dr. J. H. Tilden, quoted in Herbert M. Shelton, *Fasting Can Save Your Life* (Tampa: Natural Hygiene Press, 1981), 36. Although I don't agree with all of Dr. Tilden's views, statements like this are very common in his books and articles regarding preventative healthcare.
5. Quoted from https://www.genome.gov/genetics-glossary/Telomere.
6. Here is a helpful short clip from Ben Horne, MD: https://www.youtube.com/watch?v=s8AbGq2oG1Y and another one from Dr. LeGrand here: https://www.youtube.com/watch?v=_KI3Pmn1Egw

BE ON GUARD IN THESE TWO AREAS

1. Dr. Joel Fuhrman comes to this same conclusion regarding meat and sugar. He breaks it down here: https://www.youtube.com/watch?v=uXMzWkzqkao.
2. If you're searching for God, please take time to read the full sermon by C.H. Spurgeon here https://www.blueletterbible.org/Comm/spurgeon_charles/sermons/0969.cfm.

STIMULANTS—ROBBING PETER AND PLUNDERING PAUL

1. Are There Risks and Benefits of Energy Drinks? https://nutritionfacts.org/video/flashback-friday-are-there-risks-and-benefits-of-energy-drinks/.

IF YOU FAIL, FALL FORWARD

1. Commonly attributed to Dr. D. H. "Dee" Groberg. If you need encouragement, find the poem online titled "The Race." It's well worth the read.

WHAT TYPE OF FAST SHOULD I DO?

1. J. Harold Smith, *Fast Your Way to Health*, published by Thomas Nelson © 1979, pgs. 23-24. He also stated the following about his twenty-eight day fast, "How did I feel? Every fiber of my sixty-five-year-old body rejoiced. I felt great! Yes, it's true there were times when, if I suddenly stood up, I would feel light headed. But the dizziness was only momentary."
2. The University of Scotland oversaw his fast for the entire period. Blood glucose levels held around 30 mg/100 ml consistently during the last eight months of the fast.

3. Although I don't agree with some of his beliefs such as evolution and drinking coffee on a fast, Dr. Jason Fung has great information for those who suffer from Type II Diabetes.
4. More can be found here https://www.healthline.com/health/eating-disorders/anorexia-vs-bulimia.
5. Here is a good paper on overcoming these eating disorders from a biblical, Christ-centered approach: http://www.quietinganoisysoul.com/downloads/anorexia-bulimia-syllabus.pdf.
6. Robert Dave Johnston, *How to Lose 40 Pounds (Or More) in 30 Days with Water Fasting*, published by Amazing Health Publishing © 2012 on Kindle. Although I don't agree with everything the author believes or promotes, this book definitely walks readers through the day-to-day struggles of water fasting and offers motivation along the way.
7. Minerals and Heart Palpitations, Sutter Health: https://www.sutterhealth.org/ask-an-expert/ask-an-expert-detail.
8. Thomas DeLauer discusses more here: https://youtu.be/9ZFDjmKXSN8.
9. Michael Klaper and Alan Goldhammer have great videos on who (and who shouldn't) fast. Also, people like Daniel Pompa and Sten Ekberg have done amazing research on this topic as well.

THE HARDEST PART OF A FAST

1. https://www.health.harvard.edu/blog/what-is-keto-flu-2018101815052#.
2. Choose a powder that has healthy, organic plant-based ingredients and does not contain GMOs, synthetic chemicals, preservatives, or sugar. There are budget friendly options, as well as expensive options that contain superfoods. Ask Karen Hix what she recommends based on your overall needs as well as your budget. Her website is https://freshwholeplantiful.com/.
3. Thomas Brooks, *The Complete Works of Thomas Brooks, Volume 2* was first published by James Nichol in 1866. The quote can be found on page 508.
4. https://www.freedomyou.com/fasting_helped_break_alcohol_addiction_freedomyou.aspx.
5. https://rodaleinstitute.org/blog/wait-organic-farmers-use-pesticides/.
6. https://www.ewg.org/research/glyphosate-hummus/.

BIBLICALLY SPEAKING, WHAT SHOULD I EAT?

1. Quotes from Dr. Caldwell Esselstyn and Ann Wigmore.
2. Watch: *Eating The Right Mix Of Veggies, Nuts And Seeds Makes The Most Effective Way To Prevent Heart Attack* at https://www.youtube.com/watch?v=uRWoJk_g8rs.
3. The Keto Guide to Water Fasting: https://ketonedbodies.com/blogs/blog/the-keto-guide-to-water-fasting.

NOTES

4. First option: https://www.drfuhrman.com/blog/64/how-plant-protein-wins-over-animal-protein.
   Second option: https://www.nomeatathlete.com/where-vegetarians-get-protein/.
   Third option: https://www.forksoverknives.com/wellness/vegan-protein-guide-athletes/.
   Fourth option: https://nutritionfacts.org/video/the-great-protein-fiasco/.
5. *Answers in Genesis* provides a well-documented chart titled "Timeline for the Flood" here https://answersingenesis.org/bible-timeline/timeline-for-the-flood/.
6. The *Eat, Fast & Live Longer BBC Documentary* has a lot of good information about this topic: https://www.youtube.com/watch?v=Ihhj_VSKiTs.
7. For those desiring more information, click here for a brief article about meat and dairy and their effects on the body: https://www.whitneyerd.com/2019/05/the-truth-about-meat-inflammation.html.
8. Dr. Joel Fuhrman comes to this same conclusion regarding meat and sugar. He breaks it down in this video, *How to Prevent Disease*, https://www.youtube.com/watch?v=uXMzWkzqkao&t=6s.
9. In case you missed it, here it is again: *Eating The Right Mix Of Veggies, Nuts And Seeds Makes The Most Effective Way To Prevent Heart Attack* at https://www.youtube.com/watch?v=uRWoJk_g8rs.
10. Informative article on the effects of fiber fighting disease and also as a great anti-inflammatory aid: https://nutritionfacts.org/video/is-fiber-an-effective-anti-inflammatory/.
11. More at https://www.ewg.org/foodnews/strawberries.php.
12. Link is here for more info: https://www.healthline.com/health/chronic-dehydration#complications.
13. https://nutritionfacts.org/video/whats-your-gut-microbiome-enterotype/.
14. https://www.nytimes.com/2005/03/17/health/childrens-life-expectancy-being-cut-short-by-obesity.html

A MUST-READ FASTING EXPERIENCE

1. https://rehabilitateyourheart.wordpress.com/2012/10/12/cool-facts-about-blood-vessels/
2. Brief exhortation at Godspeak church https://www.youtube.com/watch?v=91HgO76G4H4&t=4s

1. HOW TO REST IN TURBULENT TIMES

1. https://www.crosswalk.com/church/pastors-or-leadership/reasons-spiritual-leaders-should-rest.html.

6. TRUTH–A HILL ON WHICH TO DIE

1. Although I don't agree with everything, such as his conclusion about the gifts of the Spirit, the *MacArthur Study Bible* is a good choice. David Jeremiah, Chuck Smith, and others have great resources as well. On non-essential topics where Christian men and women disagree such as the rapture, gifts of the Spirit, Calvinism, and so on, it's best to read both sides before forming any strong opinions.

11. RESETTING YOUR SITE ON THE TARGET

1. https://www.wnd.com/2013/04/americans-snapping-by-the-millions/.

12. THIS WORD WILL SET YOU FREE

1. Richard Owen Roberts, *Repentance: The First Word of the Gospel*, published by Crossway © 2002. The quote can be found in the introduction.

13. EXPERIENCING GOD THROUGH HIS SPIRIT

1. For those desiring a deeper relationship with God, I highly recommend the book, *Deeper Experiences of Famous Christians* by James Gilchrist Lawson. It contains short biographies of believers who were radically transformed by the power of God.
2. Do you really want revival? Then listen to this sermon on The Genuine Cost of Revival: https://www.youtube.com/watch?v=zYfN3jHqek4&t=1381s

16. MONEY—SERVANT OR MASTER?

1. On March 30, 1863, Abraham Lincoln issued a historic proclamation appointing a National Fast Day.

18. IS THE WORLD INFECTING YOU?

1. Author unknown.

26. UNDERSTANDING GRACE

1. From a sermon transcript, but the exact location of the quote could not be found.

31. THERE IS ANOTHER IN THE FIRE WITH YOU

1. Sermon here: https://www.youtube.com/watch?v=Q9uWhWBXJ6M.
2. Full length article: https://shaneidleman.com/2020/09/04/there-is-another-in-the-fire-with-you/.

32. SEVEN TIPS FOR TURBULENT TIMES

1. https://shaneidleman.com/2020/03/25/overcoming-fear-conquering-chaos-10-tips-for-turbulent-times/.

33. IS YOUR BLESSING WAITING ON YOU?

1. Here is one sure sign of a false prophet: https://www.youtube.com/watch?v=VQnXzF619bE.

34. FIVE WAYS TO PREVAIL IN PRAYER

1. Watch the sermon, Travail Before You Prevail: https://www.youtube.com/watch?v=Im-KvxoK5u8.

35. TRAITS OF FALSE PROPHETS

1. The full article is here. Feel free to share it with friends and family as well as on social media: https://shaneidleman.com/2020/07/13/the-battle-for-truth-7-unmistakable-traits-of-false-prophets/.
2. Why Many Christians are Divided in America: https://www.youtube.com/watch?v=-y7m-vp-dyo&t=3s.

37. DEALING WITH DEPRESSION AND MENTAL ILLNESS

1. Watch the short video here outlining these same points: https://www.youtube.com/watch?v=dYsjHEqW520
2. https://shaneidleman.com/2019/09/16/depression-and-mental-illness-5-things-you-need-to-know/.
3. Dr. Yuri Nikolayev, a psychiatrist at the University of Moscow, treated schizophrenics with water fasts for twenty-five to thirty days. This was followed by eating healthy foods for thirty days. Seventy percent of his patients remained free from symptoms for the duration of the six-year study. The health benefits of fasting are incredible.

39. SURVIVING THE ANOINTING

1. Watch the sermon, Surviving the Anointing, here: https://www.youtube.com/watch?v=iCjntehxoRM. David Ravenhill also wrote an exceptional book by the same title that I highly recommend.
2. Article here: https://shaneidleman.com/2018/12/13/7-lessons-from-samson-surviving-the-anointing/.
3. Listen to more here about waiting time not being wasted time: https://www.youtube.com/watch?v=pW-u6Apso3c&feature=youtu.be.
4. To get back on track, simply cry out, "Oh, God, remember me." This cry God will hear. Watch this sermon clip to be encouraged in this area: https://www.youtube.com/watch?v=rtZdGNtUzPo.

40. WHY REVIVAL IS AMERICA'S ONLY HOPE!

1. Article link: https://shaneidleman.com/2021/03/22/why-revival-is-americas-only-hope/.
2. https://jonathanturley.org/2021/03/19/father-arrested-after-continuing-to-call-his-child-she-after-court-ordered-gender-transition-treatments/.
3. The True Cost of Revival sermon: https://www.youtube.com/watch?v=zYfN3jHqek4&t=1385s.

APPENDIX: MY DAILY FASTING BREAKDOWN

1. The YouTube link is here: https://youtu.be/WIrY-4kK9I4.
   GodTube here: https://www.godtube.com/watch/?v=YZY7DLNX.
   Rumble here: https://rumble.com/vh1y4t-be-encouraged-by-my-30-day-fasting-journey.html.

2. *Why Revival is America's Only Hope* can be found here: https://shaneidleman.com/2021/03/22/why-revival-is-americas-only-hope/.
3. Two powerful songs: https://youtu.be/fTTxJHu7shw and https://youtu.be/E1KoUxTqxjw.
4. The article is here: https://shaneidleman.com/2021/03/26/a-battle-cry-for-a-dead-church/.

Printed in Great Britain
by Amazon